Lecture Notes in Medical Informatics

Lecture Notes in Medical Informatics

Edited by D. A. B. Lindberg and P. L. Reichertz

20

Sibylle Biefang
Wolfgang Köpcke
Martin A. Schreiber

Manual for the Planning and Implementation of Therapeutic Studies

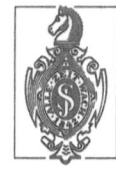

Springer-Verlag
Berlin Heidelberg New York 1983

Authors

Sibylle Biefang
Internationales Institut für wissenschaftliche Zusammenarbeit e.V.
Schloß Reisensburg, Bürgermeister-Joh.-Müller-Str. 1, 8870 Günzburg

Wolfgang Köpcke
Martin A. Schreiber
Institut für Medizinische Informationsverarbeitung, Statistik
und Biomathematik der Ludwig-Maximilians-Universität
Marchioninistr. 15, 8000 München 70

ISBN 978-3-540-11979-1   ISBN 978-3-642-93237-3 (eBook)
DOI: 10.1007/978-3-642-93237-3

Originally published by Springer-Verlag Berlin Heidelberg New York

2145/3140-543210

Foreword

The German edition of this manual appeared in 1979. Its main objective then was to extend help to those engaged in multicentric therapeutic studies, especially with respect to the "Federal Government's Program on Promoting Research and Development in the Service of Health".

Experience with therapeutic studies in the Federal Republic of Germany showed that considerable problems as to methods and implementation of such studies exist. The manual was an attempt to present current methodological knowledge and the experience obtained from completed studies in the light of the international literature. No radically new methodology was produced; however, the information representing the state-of-the art, which is widely scattered up to now, has been compiled.

For the American edition of this manual a few changes have been made. These concern especially the literature where references to German unpublished manuscripts were omitted.

The authors wish to thank Dr. Andreas Jaffé for the translation, and Evelyn Birke who typewrited the lecture-notes manuscript.

Günzburg and Munich   Sibylle Biefang
November 1981   Wolfgang Köpcke
                                                       Martin A. Schreiber

Contents

1. Methods of Therapeutic Studies

Statistical methods and their application have become an integral part
of scientific medicine and its quest for knowledge of therapeutic pro-
gress (Cornfield 1976; Meier 1975). However, applied statistical methods still appear to many doctors to constitute an estrangement of medicine in thought and action.

Clinical therapeutic trials and their planning as a prerequisite to
statistical analysis are no invention of our time. The heightened con-
sciousness of the necessity of methodology and statistical thinking in
clinical medicine may be of latter date, but it is easy to show that
this belongs to an older tradition. We may cite as one example standing
for many Sir Austin Bradford HILL's book (Hill 1966), which has appeared
again and again in repeated editions for forty years, and has propounded
the basic principles of the planning of clinical trials; its validity
is the same as at the outset.

Scientific medicine requires the methods of science and its mode of
gaining knowledge. This includes exact observation and abstract analysis of the observed in seeking causal relationships.

Statements are the more certain, the greater the degree of exactness
and formality of the observations performed. This is true of the quality of data. Omissions in this area cannot be made good by the most re-
fined statistical and mathematical techniques of analysis (Gordis 1979).
Experiment is the most formal type of observation.

In biology, which is concerned with living matter, experiments cannot
be set out as unambiguously as in physics. The experimental layout involving the enforcing of constancy of all influencing parameters cannot
be totally achieved. Hence, the multiplicity of possible reactions makes
for great ranges of variation. However, experimental quality can be
achieved by adhering to certain rules in planning and layout of experiments (Harris 1970).

Therapeutic studies - i.e., experimental clinical trials - are motivated
by medical necessity including the obligation to critically evaluate
existing forms of therapy and to develop new and better ones.

1.1. Terminology

The multiplicity in the designation of studies found in the literature
and also in some advertisements may lead to confusion or at least some
measure of insecurity.

Experimental – non-experimental	All studies may be divided, according to the respective methods chosen, in "experimental" and "non-experimental" ones. Further differentiation may be added by choosing between the opposites prospective and retrospective. We call a study experimental, in which the causal nexus is manipulated; however, the decisive criterion for the label "experimental" is an experimental layout, in which all influencing parameters, i.e., the sum of the boundary conditions, are kept constant and are thus "controlled" during the trial. This is achieved by randomization.
	Only certain influencing parameters are changed, all other conditions remaining equal. For the change in the result, the above parameter manipulation is, according to conventional usage, causal.
Prospective – retrospective	Conclusions are termed prospective, if they originate in causes at some point in time and are drawn from their effects observed along the time axis. Retrospective conclusions are drawn from observed effects backwards in time toward the antecedent causes.
Prolective – retrolective	Data and information are usually acquired parallel to one of these two directions of view. Therefore, the terms "prospective" and "retrospective" are also used in data acquisition. There may be confusion when the direction of conclusion opposes that of data acquisition, if this fact is not made clear. For example, one could deduce effects from causes (i.e., prospectively), but obtain information from archived data and anamneses pointing backward (retrospectively) into the past. The reverse situation obtains, whenever manifest effects (disease) are

put down to causes (i.e., retrospectively), but the information is gathered prospectively by register.

In order to differentiate these two processes, FEINSTEIN (1973) has proposed using the technical terms "prolective" and "retrolective" for purposes of data acquisition[+).

Experimental studies

For therapeutic studies, such strictly experimental conditions obtain only in controlled clinical trials (Atkins 1966; Cornfield, Haenszel 1960; Peto et al. 1976/77; Überla 1975). In epidemiological research, an interventional study is called experimental if methods are used ensuring the above-mentioned constancy of boundary parameters (McMahon, Pugh 1970).

Observational studies

All other study types not conforming to the strict formal requirement of control of all influencing paramters by randomization are called
- cohort studies : prospective, non-randomized observational studies,
and
- case-control studies: retrospective investigations.

Names of studies

In the above system, all studies can find their place, even if this is not immediately evident from their titles, as these may stem from organizational aspects (multicentre, open/blind, cross-sectional, longitudinal, etc.) or point to an analytical method (sequential, cross-over). Such names of studies are used to accentuate certain methods of solving specific problems.

[+) The usage of the terms is still fluctuating and not yet consolidated, which is especially true of "controlled". If only a control group is kept during a trial, this minimum prerequisite of trial planning should not receive this label. Thus, "controlled" would become an unambiguous synonym for "randomized".

1.2. Experimental Design

Before we look into individual types of studies, we will describe the
facts relating to all types of trial planning. - Knowledge is, in this
context, the finding out of differences by comparing; this formula may
be used for rationally reproducible knowledge, without denying that
other paths to knowledge may exist in other branches of science (e.g.,
the heuristic method).

To find out a possibly existing difference, this must become visible.
The purpose of a question is to sharpen and focus the field of vision
in question. The structure of an experiment suited to a given question
is expressed in an experimental design. This is the formal framework
necessarily preceding the formulated problem. Differences can only be
shown by appropriate comparisons; in the experimental design, the necessary preconditions for comparability are created.

A number of experimental designs has been developed covering a wide
range of problems; these fit many problems in medicine, but not all -
and some only after modification (Armitage 1971; Cochran, Cox 1957;
Hölzel, Überla 1978; Peto et al. 1976/77). The great number of statistical methods of analysis in the strict sense of the term presupposes experimental designs and covers the "differences", including their quanti-
fication and their significance.

The assessment of such rationally reproducible pieces of knowledge and
their application in practical decision-making transcends the area of
experimental design and leads us to other areas of methodology, such as
decision theory (Cornfield 1976; Lindley 1975; Raiffa 1968; Susser 1973
and 1977).

Problem
formulation

The question
field

The formulated problem is the guideline for the
entire experimental set-up. It may appear super-
fluous to point to this fact, but experience bears
out that this is justified. The existence of a ha-
zily defined general question is never sufficient.
It is, on the contrary, necessary to define and
formulate the problem in full details, and in writing; all such details must be sufficiently clarified by discussion among the scientists involved

in the project. Generalized problem formulations, which in fact contain a manifold of sub-questions, must be broken down, if anything more is expected of the result of the study than an equally general (and vague) statement for an answer. This necessitates fixing the decision variables constituting the ultimate answer in advance.

A small number of sub-questions

We must oppose the tendency to attempt to answer a great number of questions by a single study. We prefer using simple, few and unambiguous question formulations: these furnish more definite answers.

Whether a given formulation is concrete and detailed enough, is measurable by checking whether possible and foreseeable outcomes are anticipated and rationally structured and are listed in the records of the study.

Comparisons
Casuistry

Even when a comparison seems to be missing, it is indispensable. Single-case studies - casuistry - seem to have no need of comparisons. However, the special properties shown for single cases are found only with reference to typical cases, other ones and cases in general. Hence, a comparison is implied in the special features of the studied case.

The control group

Thus, even a new method of therapy may, without a control group in the usual sense, be compared to earlier results (historical control), and be consequently assessed. An example of this is the advent of penicillin therapy. However, this method is restricted to exceptions of this type. It is obvious that such comparisons are only qualitative. For stringent outcome statements, it is indispensable to keep a control group for direct comparison. Reports on successful therapies which refer only to these without using comparisons are worthless, as they may show nothing more than the natural course of the disease and/or the recovery therefrom. In contradistinction to the above example and other

known causal therapies (such as substitution of
singular metabolic defects), where there is a
single causal chain in evidence, most therapeutic
studies are situated in an "area of therapeutic
indifference", where the problem consists in show-
ing either
- therapeutic effectiveness as such,
or
- therapeutic superiority to conventional therapy.
A criterion of therapeutic equality may be set out
as a given range of difference or pre-set deviation
to or from previous results.

Comparability

In order to make comparisons, comparability must
demonstrably exist, or be created. This property
is subdivided in
- structural equality: the equality of the object
  of investigation regarding structural features
  such as age, sex, etc. and the influencing parameters (boundary conditions) involved;
- observational equality: that of counting, measurement, weighing, judging and diagnosis;
- procedural equality: that of the procedures administered or followed.

First, we must add some remarks concerning the last
of these points. All other comment is made on the
other points, i.e., structural and observational
equality. Differences in the type and frequency of
examinations, doctors' attention, place, time, etc.
can materially influence the attitude of patients
to their illness and thus affect the assessment of
the results of therapy, as long as these do not
solely consist of laboratory data. We must also
mention the motivated cooperation of the patient
with treatment (compliance) in this connection.

Generalization

For procedural equality, the classical KOLLER
(1975) classification substitutes representational
equality. This refers to the general transferabi-
lity of the results obtained by the study group to
all patients having the same indication. However,

a therapeutic study cannot achieve representation
of all possible patients (including future ones).
We must stress that all inferences can only be valid for their inductive base. Applications beyond
such base to other patients necessitate checking
whether these subjects meet the criteria for this
base of the original therapeutic study. Transfer-
ence of results is then made by analogy. A necessary prerequisite to this is a sufficient description of said base in the publications used.

The study
protocoll

All details of experimental design, implementation
and evaluation must become part of the study protocol. This must be created in writing during the
design phase and not be only a current "log-book"
or a retrospective write-up. The study protocol is
a guideline and a check for decisions made during
the entire study; such decisions arise from a process of discussion. These guidelines are also the
solid foundation for possible modifications which
may become necessary during the study itself.

Bipartition of
the study
protocol

With some very columinous study protocols, it may
be useful to subdivide the protocol in
- an experimental design containing the fundamen-
   tal, i.e., the overall strategy,
and in
- an experimental schedule containing the details
   of implementation and procedures for diagnosis,
   laboratory work and related matters; this is
   used to inform and motivate the personnel involved.

Voluminous study protocols are almost bound to be
created in multicentre studies. However, even when
working with complex organizations, the problem
formulation and the protocol should be kept as
simple and lucid as possible.

With such a bipartition of the study protocol, the
first part may be thought to represent the structural equality envisioned, whereas the second part is

allocated to the conservation of observational
equality. Thus, the first part specifies particu-
lars of structural features such as the indication,
the contraindications, the diagnosis in operation-
alized elements, the efficacy criteria, etc.. The
second part is intended to help ensure observational equality and contains standardizations and ob-
jectifications of the "impressions" to be gained
and regulations for all the activities envisioned.

Observations should, if possible, be made by the
same doctors and other personnel. In long-term
studies, this is not achievable due to natural
personnel turnover. A detailed experimental schedule can help toward minimizing such effects on
continuity.

The necessity to detail an experimental design
down to the minutiae of a schedule becomes especially obvious with multicentre studies, with
differently organized and equipped hospitals participation (Selbmann 1978).

Questionnaire   The questionnaires and the directions for their
completion are an integral part of the experiment-
al schedule and make, by standardizing the data,
for completeness and equality of observation. Thus,
the questionnaires should be regarded as an opera-
tionalized instrument of the experimental design.

The quality   The determination of the proper number of cases
of a study   depends on the magnitude of the difference in
effect to be observed; the smaller this difference
is, the greater the number of cases required. It
is an objective of statistical experimental design
to manage with the smallest possible "sufficient"
number of cases. The number of cases involved may
be estimated according to certain preconditions
(Meydrech, Kupper 1978; Schlesselman 1974). The
quality of a study is not determined by "fascina-
tingly" large numbers, but by the care invested in
its design and by the exactness of its implementa-

tion. Similarly, the numerical significance of
some small difference is not of decisive importance, but only the medical relevance of the fact.

Closed and open
experimental
designs

Usually, a fixed sample size is defined - a method
preferred as lending itself more readily to processing (Walter 1977).As against this, a sequential
plan (Armitage 1957; Atkins 1966) does not fix the
number of patients in advance, except for an upper
limit; the end of the study is determined by its
course. The end is reached the earlier and with
the less cases, the greater the superiority of one
of the compared therapies is, and the later (up to
the pre-fixed limit), the lesser this difference
is seen to be. Sequential procedure has also been
described in retrospective studies (Bross 1952;
O'Neil, Anello 1978).

Inclusion, exclusion and outcome criteria, concomitant features

The patient
filter

The salient features according to which patients
are selected for inclusion in the study are called
inclusion criteria; this is the indication sector.
Similarly, the list of exclusion criteria comprises
both the contraindications and features (diseases)
associated with the outcome criterion; the latter
can have adverse effects as confounding variables
(cf. blocking and matching).

Outcome
criteria

The recommendation to predetermine the smallest
possible number of outcome criteria (efficacy criteria, judgmental criteria, etc.) is just a re-
statement of the above-mentioned requirement for a
simple problem formulation. Multiplicity of judgmental criteria increases the sample size and necessitates multivariate statistical tests. Such
tests exist; however, we must check whether the
model assumptions of such tests conform to the
real situation in each case - and this must be done

for each individual study. Moreover, the interpretation of results in terms of effect by component remains a problem with a view to the final assessment of the therapies in question.

Concomitant
features

Besides the outcome criteria used for statistical testing in the classical sense of the term, a number of concomitant features must be incorporated in the observation and standardized data acquisition as further information. This enables a descriptive - not statistically testable - presentation of the entire problem to be made, and gives the background and context needed for an otherwise unsatisfactory interpretation of the dichotomous (yes/no) statements on significance yielded by the statistical tests. Often, such features are described in evaluations by means of "descriptive significance" not computed by tests in the strict sense of the word, but by an analogous procedure.

Blind observations
Soft data

In order to attain as independent and unbiased observations and assessments as possible, the observations may be made "blind". This is to be recommended in all cases in which an important part of the information to be gathered consists of so-called "soft" data, i.e., subjective judgments by patients and doctors. In such situations, a negative effect on the quality of the assessment is to be feared due to inwitting preference or prejudice, which is readily eliminated by a "blind" procedure. In simple blind studies, the patients do not know which subject gets which medicine; the double-blind procedure also excludes doctors and medical personnel from this knowledge; the "triple-blind" mode also keeps the methodologist and statisticians involved equally in the dark. The blind procedure is nothing but a tool used to ensure unbiased observations, and does not of itself justify calling a study "controlled".

1.3. Types of Studies

Besides the requisites mentioned in the foregoing, we must list the
principles of biostatistical research introduced 50 years ago by FISHER.
These are :
- repetition
- blocking
- allocation by chance.
These are part of the process of exploration of the natural range of
variation, and are used to control known and unknown influence and interference parameters. As these elements are used without restrictions only
in controlled clinical studies, they will be discussed under this head-
ing.

<u>The controlled</u> <u>clinical study</u>	This type of study is analogous in design to a scientific experiment, in which influencing para- meters are varied according to a plan while all other variables are kept constant. Changes in the result are thus causally related to the variations in the onset conditions. This is a prospective method, i.e., deduction from cause to effect follows the course of time (as against the opposite temporal order of retrospective studies).
	In general, the system between the input and out- put - the organism(s) - must be regarded as a "black box", in which an unknown number of causal processes operate, so that simple causality cannot be assumed.
Repetition	Repeating measurements and observations under stan- dard conditions gives us information on the size of the error involved, of the variation of a given quantity (such as daily range), and of the variation between individual subjects. Besides instrument-re- lated errors in measurement, there exist inter- and intra-individual variations. This (overall) varia- bility evidenced by repetition is an important quan- tity bearing on the precision of subsequently com- puted statistics.
	The number of subjects (n) is also a measure of re- petition. n must be greater than the number of ne-

cessary observational criteria (c); according to a rule of thumb, n must be at least three times c, or $n \geq 3c$ (Fink 1978).

Known influencing parameters; blocking

Besides the main influencing parameter, such as a new therapy, there always exist a large number of other influencing parameters with effect on the outcome; these factors can "falsify" the result in one way or another. Each influencing parameter can, depending on the problem, become "interference". Although we try, by providing for comparability (as set out above), to attribute differences in the compared groups solely to the manipulated differences in the main influencing parameter we know that, as far as biological research is concerned, an unknown set of other influencing parameters remains and cannot be eliminated.

If these are known as influencing parameters (risk factors, compounding diseases, supplementary therapies, etc.) of which effects and interactions are to be analyzed and incorporated into the study, a blocking (stratification) procedure is initiated; this produces subgroups with greater internal homogeneity, i.e., the intra-block variation is intended to become smaller than the inter-block one.

Blocking eliminates the error produced by certain interference variables on the outcome inasmuch as this error becomes known and may consequently be eliminated from the overall result.

For practical reasons, only a limited number of interference parameters can be controlled by stratification. As a rule, all important influencing parameters must be taken into account. Thus, stratified analysis is rendered possible, even if no systematic blocking was performed at the outset; if such blocking was done, subdivision into further subgroups may be possible.

Unknown
influences and
randomization

After the above-mentioned precautions, we still
have to contend with a great number of usually unknown influencing parameters, which may distort
the result by creating spurious differences or
masking genuine ones. The requisite conditions of
an experimental arrangement are fulfilled only if,
with the exception of the principal influencing
parameter, all other boundary conditions are rendered equal in the groups being compared. For the
remaining, uncontrollable parameters, this is
achieved by randomizaiton, i.e., a strict allocation by chance only.

Randomization is recognized as the only way to
eliminate a practically unlimited number of unknown
influencing factors, as these are evenly distribu-
ted with respect to the groups or strata, so that
any difference in the outcome may not be attributed
to an otherwise possible unequal distribution of
such factors. The randomization procedure must
follow a genuine pure-chance mechanism and be stipulated in the study record. This is a precaution
against "personally" motivated allocation of patients to specific therapies, a procedure entail-
ing conscious or unconscious preferences and therefore rendering the achievement of comparability impossible.

Hence, randomization is called for where a choice
filter has created a "zone of therapeutic indifference" of the therapies to be compared. If a patient
is eligible for the study after passing the filter
of in- and exclusion criteria and has been allocated to his stratum (if applicable), randomization
then decides on the therapy he receives.

If randomized allocation is provided for in the
design of a study, one should not settle for any
surrogate. So-called systematic random allocation
according to even/odd data of admission, birthdate,
admission number or the initial letter of names of
patients is much less reliable without having the

advantage of being easier to administer.

Preconditions for randomization

In the clinical setting, randomization meets with considerable difficulties, mostly for reasons of professional ethics. An important prerequisite to randomization of clinical trials on human subjects is the condition that no reliable knowledge of Therapy A being definitely better than Therapy B may exist, when A and B are therapies to be tested. The same holds true for important side-effects. If this condition is not fulfilled, randomization cannot be tolerated for reasons of medical ethics : a group of patients may not be purposely denied the better treatment. Thus, "equivalence" of the therapies to be studied must be in evidence according to current knowledge. The doctors involved in the therapy must also "know" that A and B are equivalent, as nobody may demand from a doctor that he uses a therapy on his patients which he feels to be inferior. This would not only be an onerous constraint running counter to the current legal tenet of ultimate responsibility and therapeutic freedom of the individual doctor; moreover, a source of errors would come into existence which would be difficult to assess, as this situation would affect the clinical opinion regarding each case in the pre-selection stage, and thus lead to severe selection bias with attendant falsification of the outcome.

Random allocation and medical ethics

Random allocation in controlled clinical trials has led to discussion of the ethical propriety of such action among specialists and also in the public. Critics question not the methodological correctness, but the conflicting of social versus individual rights and values. We cannot do justice to this problem in our present framework.

However, the following statement may be made from the definition: only constant outset conditions confer on a study the quality of experimental evidence. If this is achieved without randomization, the burden of proof in this respect is on the persons responsible for conducting the individual study in question.

Clinical studies are hence entitled to the label "experimental", if they are controlled in that they are randomized. These two terms may be regarded as synonymous. For reasons of honesty and terminological clarity, the above-mentioned label should be used only in such cases.

Prospective, non-randomized observational studies

Formal requirements

Whenever the rigorous methodological requirement of randomization cannot be fulfilled (for any reason whatsoever), but the other principles and preconditions, such as the existence of a control group, exactly defined structural and observational equality, repetition and stratification, are adhered to, the type of study involved is called a non-randomized prospective observational study, as causality is being observed during the course of time (Cochran 1965 and 1963; McKinlay 1975).

For example, randomization is hardly feasible if a surgical team used to a therapeutic process is forced to modify the same from time to time. Similarly random allocation may be difficult or impossible in psychotherapy and social therapy, if therapy suited to different individuals has to be applied under widely differing outset conditions: the effective causes to be considered regarding such therapies are not only easily definable drugs, but also the effect of the personality and persuasive power of the therapist, which latter may be the greater factor in the therapeutic process.

Examples of studies

Non-randomized studies have been described - inter alia - in the field of cancer chemotherapy (Gehan, Freireich 1974). Other examples are epidemiological cohort studies, which, as long-term projects, often keep very voluminous registers. Studies of this type include the Framingham study (Gordon et al. 1959), the Boston Collaborative Drug Surveillance Program (1974), and studies designed to elucidate risks of large general populations, such as the Heidelberg-Wiesloch-Eberbach project as a part of the WHO studies on cardiac infarction (Nüssel et al. 1975). The same holds true of drug monitoring for drugs already marketed and for follow-up studies, in which new drugs are observed among other factors in the complex "natural" environment of practical medical service (Friebel 1975; Jick 1977).

For all non-randomized studies, an attempt must be made to uncover all relevant influencing parameters and their effects, and to "eliminate" them by enforcing sufficient structural equality of the control groups. The former is effected by stratification, and the latter is understood with respect to the distortion of results, not to the primary effects of the factors on the objects studied (Greenland 1977).

Retrospective observational studies (case-control studies)

There is some measure of contrast between case-control studies and controlled clinical studies. Firstly, the temporal direction of logical conclusion is "reversed", i.e., retrospective: it is attempted to find the cause from the effect looking backwards in time (Cornfield 1956; Feinstein 1973; Mantel, Haenszel 1959). Secondly, randomization can be used only in certain cases as a tool for equalization of influencing parameters.

Relative risk

The result computed in such studies is, besides the significance of an overall difference between the groups compared, the "relativ risk". This is the ratio of exposure to defined risk factors ("risk indicators") of the case group versus the control group. This "relative risk" (odds ratio, cross ratio, etc.) is an estimator or index for the potency of the relationship computed as the quotient

of the two exposure ratios (Breslow 1976; Cornfield,
Haenszel 1960; McMahon, Pugh 1970; Miettinen 1970
and 1976; Seigel, Greenhouse 1973). For positive
associations, such as smoking with lung cancer,
this quotient exceeds unity ($>$1); for negative
associations, such as cardiac infarction with aspirin ingestion, it is less than unity ($<$1). The
quotient approaches unity for progressively weaker
relationships. For large-scale representative studies of populations, this index becomes the measure
of the relative risk for specific diseases. For
case-control studies, it is an estimator for the
exposure-induced risk for cases (McMahon, Pugh
1970). The question whether such results reflect
causality or non-causal correlations remains un-
answered at this stage of research.

Generating
hypotheses

Interpretation of the results of case-control studies must proceed in the context of the general
scientific knowledge in the field in question.
Stringency of the relationships found is conspi-
cuously missing. We are faced with the task of generating hypotheses, as long as no pre-existing
hypotheses are to be confirmed (or disproved). In
some cases, the results of retrospective case-control studies may be corroborated only by an experimental prospective arrangement; however, it may be
that such research were to become unnecessary or
ethically unviable on account of the magnitude of
an effect shown with a sufficient degree of reliability (e.g., impairments due to thalidomide).

Advantages/
disadvantages

Case-control studies have the advantage that they
may produce results in a relatively short period
of time which can be very important for public
health uses (for example, the aforementioned thalidomide defects). The time saving is a result of
making an indefinitely long observation period
available for the present, as the retrospective
method deals only with events in elapsed time (as
against prospective studies, in which the events
must be waited for, and sometimes for years or de-

cades). However, projecting past observations into the present has disadvantages too: the observations may be inexact and incomplete; this has adverse effects on structural and observational equality.

Erroneous classification

This problem makes for erroneous classification (false positive and false negative) in the process of allocation of risk, which, in turn, may materially change the resulting index of relative risk (Bross 1954). Thus, the main objection to case-control studies is to the insufficient and/or questionable comparability of the two groups (i.e., selection bias). A number of methods and regulations have been described to eliminate such errors as far as possible by testing for them before the analysis proper is begun (Breslow et al. 1978; Prentice 1976).

Matching

In order to achieve greater structural comparability, the method of matching is used (Fischer, Patil 1974; Hardy, White 1971; Holford et al. 1978; McKinlay 1977; Miettinen 1968; Worcester 1964). This is essentially the pairing-off of cases, which is analogous to stratification in prospective studies. Matching lessens the overall variability to obtain more homogeneity and greater statistical efficiency (Cochran 1953). Besides frequency matching, in which pairs of groups are formed, individual matching is an important method: either several controls are matched to a case, or the special method of one-to-one matching is used, which has the advantage of appreciably facilitated analysis (Bross 1969; Miettinen 1969 and 1970; Pike et al. 1975).

The controls for each case are selected according to existing structural features such as sex, age, race, socio-economic status, parity, etc.. In addition to such matching criteria, known and relevant influencing parameters are included in the process of forming matched pairs. The latter receive special attention if such parameters are associated with the outcome criterion under study and/or with

the suspected cause, and may consequently falsify
the result of the study if they are unevenly distri-
buted. Matched criteria themselves cannot be evalu-
ated.

Overmatching

This is the error ensuing whenever a factor is used
for matching pairs which is part of the direct causal chain between the outcome and its suspected
cause (i.e., risk factor). Such mistakes lead to
falsely negative conclusions from the computed result (McMahon, Pugh 1970). This experience is evidence for the fact that matching as a method is not
free of problems, and that the criteria matched for
must be very carefully selected (Hardy, White 1971).
This situation exists because the number of such
criteria is limited. Moreover, with each additional
criterion, the difficulty of finding suitable controls with the same combination of features grows.
For reasons of feasibility, the number of matching
criteria is limited to 7 or 10 (at most). Differing
techniques for matching discrete and continuous
variables have been described.

Matching and
the number
of cases

Cases for which no suitable match is found must be
eliminated. For an increasing number of matching
criteria, the loss of cases also rises, especially
if the matching is to be effective (Althauser, Rubin
1970). Furthermore, the reserve from which the controls are taken must be several times larger than
the planned number of cases. For 10 matching variables, the ratio is 5:1 - 6:1 (Cochran 1965; Freedman 1950; McKinlay 1977). Tables are given in the
literature for estimating numbers of cases and of
possible matches (McKinlay 1974; Meydrech, Kupper
1978; Schlesselman 1974).

Registers

The existence of comprehensive registers facilitates
forming matched pairs in particular and improves
comparability in retrospective studies in general,
as the variables were compiled prospectively (in
this case, prolectively) while the register in
question was kept. Registers are generally used for

prospective follow-up and are at the same time the basis for accurate case-control studies. An example is the negative correlation found between acetyl-salicylic acid and myocardial infarction, which was first shown in a case-control study of the Boston Collaborative Drug Surveillance Program (1974).

Case-Control studies are not usually applied as primary tests of the efficacy of new therapies, but are the method best suited to the monitoring of drugs and other types of therapy, especially when checking for long-term (side-)effects (Lindley 1971).

1.4. Steps in Drug Testing

The testing of a drug throughout the four stages usually defined is described as an example of the differing application of the study types referred to above (Gross, Inman 1977; Staak, Weiser 1978). Legal aspects are not discussed here.

Phase I
During this phase, a broad spectrum of questions exists as to pharmacokinetics, pharmacodynamics, metabolism, toxicity, dosage, side-effects, toler-ance, etc. (Imhof 1973; Wolf 1975). The drug is tested on a small number of subjects - usually vo-lunteers. There is no randomization and no control group. Randomization is not called for in this first stage of preliminary testing: "It would obscure the purpose and delay the action" (Gehan, Freireich 1974, p. 199).

However, the necessity for comparison and for de-tailed planning remains (Walter 1977). The compari-sons are between the "before" and "after" states of the individual subjects, who are construed as re-presenting single blocks or strata. The transfer of conclusions from single cases to other persons is made by analogy and not statistically. With a larger number of subjects and strata (dose, sex, etc.), stratification plans (e.g. Latin squares) can be used. Phase I, the tolerance trial, corresponds closely with a non-randomized prospective observational study.

Phase II and
Phase III

Phase II, the effectiveness trial, is likewise implemented for carefully selected subjects or patients whose number is somewhat larger (about 50); the tolerated dose is tested for effectiveness regarding the indications envisioned (Kleinsorge, 1975; Überla 1973). This stage and the subsequent Phase III of broad clinical trials follow the experimental design of controlled, i.e., randomized clinical trials.

Phase IV

If a drug is marketed and not used only in clinics, the attendant monitoring is referred to as Phase IV. The purpose of this activity is gathering of experience as to side-effects and additional indications, and may be called a long-term experiment (Friebel 1975). The most suitable methods used in this stage are non-randomized prospective and retrospective observational studies (Jick 1977; Jick, Vessey 1978; Shapiro, Slone 1977).

2. Checklist for the Planning, Implementation and Evaluation of Therapeutic Studies

The aim of this chapter is to draw up a checklist for the salient points
to be considered during the design, implementation and evaluation of
therapeutic studies. This checklist is intended to enable the doctors,
scientists,and sponsoring institutions involved in these activities
to examine a study proposal as to completeness. There will, of course,
always be some therapeutic studies in which not all points mentioned
in this checklist must be taken into account; however, even for such
cases, the catalogue set out in the following may fulfil an important
purpose: to remind all involved of the reasons why certain requirements
of the checklist were disregarded. The aspects set out in Ch. 2.1.,
"Planning of Experiments" are relevant mainly for controlled clinical
trials, whereas the principles formulated in the later sections remain
valid for nearly all types of therapeutic studies.

The subsequent remarks mainly follow JESDINSKY (1978), the articles by
ÜBERLA et al. (Hölzel, Überla 1978; Köpcke, Überla 1978; Selbmann 1978)
and the recommendations, fact sheets and question catalogues of reports
of the WORLD HEALTH ORGANIZATION (1968/1975). Further comprehensive
material on the entire field of therapeutic studies has appeared in v.
EICKSTEDT and GROSS (1975), FÜLGRAFF and KEWITZ (1979), GOOD (1976),
HARRIS and FITZGERALD (1970), JOHNSON and JOHNSON (1977), KUEMMERLE
(1978), MARTINI et al. (1968), and STAAK and WEISER (1978). Further
literature on special problems is referred to in connection with the
individual points of the checklist discussed below.

2.1. Planning of Experiments

Current status
of knowledge
in the field

The current status of knowledge in the field to be
studied must be comprehensively stated with reference
to information gathered and studies completed to
date. This inventory should include information on
previous and current work done by the applicants,
a review of the existing domestic and foreign literature and of the results obtained by contacts with
other specialists (Johnson, Johnson 1977; Wade 1970).

Formulation
of the
problem

An important step in planning a therapeutic study
is the exact formulation of the question to be
answered by the study. Problems typical for clinical

studies are the following (Jesdinsky 1978; Johnson, Johnson 1977; World Health Organization 1968 and 1975):

- proof that any therapy is beneficial with regard to the natural course of a given disease
- comparison of therapeutic effectiveness of repeated applications
- demonstration of dose-effect relationships, and, where applicable, comparison of such relationships for different therapies
- testing for constancy of therapeutic efficacy in repeated applications
- assessment of combinations of therapies
- comparison of therapeutic efficacy for different groups of patients.

It is important to limit the number of questions and to formulate each of them in precise and simple terms. This has, however, a drawback in that the resulting answers are confined to specific situations. On the other hand, too complex problem formulations may make it difficult to give any positive answer at all after completion of the study.

Comparative therapy

Clinical studies without comparative therapy do not allow conclusive answers to be found. In principle, five types of comparison are possible:

- Comparison of the therapy under trial to a group not treated at all. However, this is not feasible as a rule for ethical and legal reasons.
- Comparison of the therapy with placebo, which is the best check for spontaneous changes in the course of illnesses and for therapy-independent events. However, ethical considerations often militate against this type of comparison.
- Comparison between the therapy under study and the standard treatment, wherein the latter is regarded as constituting a control group. This procedure is necessary in all cases of serious illness in which the standard treatment is positively known to be effective.
- Comparison between two or more different applications of the same therapy, such as differing doses

and/or time sequences of administration of a sub-
stance under study and dissimilar organizational
and administrative structures, etc..
- Comparison between early and late effects of the
  same treatment.
These five basic types of comparison may be com-
bined to form complex experimental designs. However,
the design should be kept as simple as possible,
especially in multicentre studies, in order to ensure feasibility (Chalmers et al. 1972; Liberman
1961; Schindel 1967).

Control groups

Differing control groups may be kept according to
the outcome and influence variables and operational
aspects (Hölzel, Überla 1978; Liberman 1961; McKin-
ley 1977). The most simple model is the group comparison, in which the groups of patients once formed
are treated differently. A special type of this
procedure is working with matched pairs, with patients matched as set out above undergoing differing therapies. Individual comparisons should be
mentioned in this connection: in these, each individual is his own control: the left side may be
compared to the right, or later treatments with
earlier ones. This latter type of comparison is
subject to constraints due to the natural course
of diseases and to carry-over effects. Such effects
may be lessened by administering placebos between
treatments.

Randomization

Whenever two or more therapies are to be compared
during a study, we must make efforts toward elimi-
nating all differences between the groups involved
except the difference in their treatment.

To achieve such comparability (structural equality),
the tool of randomization is used, in that the therapies are allocated to the patients by chance (Byar
et al. 1976; Deeley 1966; Feinstein 1973; Kempthorne 1977; Zelen 1977). Randomization is utilized
to distribute all conceivable interference factors

which would otherwise make any comparison of therapies impossible, as small as possible. Randomization is realized at best by using a table of random numbers (Documenta Geigy 1975). Other allocation modes such as by birthdate or date of admission cannot be recommended, as these may induce or imply conscious or unconscious errors by the doctors carrying out the treatments.

Some authors have recommended, as an alternative to randomized comparisons, working with retrospective data on a standard therapy, i.e., using "historical controls". This has the advantage that all patients included in a study get the new therapy which the scientists advocating it believe or hope to be better than the conventional one. However, the great disadvantage of such historical controls is the fact that one can usually not be sure of comparability being maintained between the patient groups and between the methods used in evaluation.

Historical controls and other non-randomized modes of allocation are discussed especially by CORNFIELD (1976), GEHAN and FREIREICH (1974), POCOCK (1976), RUDNICK and CAPIZZI (1977), and by WEINSTEIN (1974).

Stratification   Stratification or blocking is used to eliminate variables with a known effect on therapeutic success, such as age and sex. This may be accomplished by randomizing only the members of one block or stratum. Whereas unknown interference factors can be controlled by randomization, we should eliminate known influencing variables by stratification. This makes for a gain in accuracy, which is found only if the scatter between the experimental units is significantly greater than between the strata (Feinstein 1973; Green, Byar 1978; Zelen 1974).

Establishing the number of cases   Establishing the required number of cases for a therapeutic study is never only a statistical problem, but also a clinical and organizational one in

each individual case. For a given plan covering a
study, minimum numbers of cases may be estimated
under certain hypotheses. For this, the statistician needs the following advance information (Fink
1976):

- The size of the difference between the test
  group and the control group regarded as clinically relevant must be established in advance.
- The variance of the outcome variable must be
  estimated.
- Distribution hypotheses must exist regarding all
  outcome variables (e.g., normal distribution).
- The probability of the error of the first (and
  sometimes also of the second) kind must be given.

For different outset conditions, we may obtain a
considerable number of different numbers of cases;
this outcome must be adjusted to fit the clinical
and organizational parameters (such as the drop-
out rate) for the therapeutic study envisioned
(Schork, Remington 1967). There are generally two
strategies to choose from with respect to establishing the method of evaluation:

- The pre-set plan, in which the numbers of cases
  are fixed in advance. For this purpose we refer
  the reader to GEORGE and DESU (1974) and to HAL-
  PERIN et al. (1968) for tables and formulae and
  to CLARK and DOWNIE (1966), and to SCHNEIDERMANN
  (1964) for nomograms presented therein.
- The sequential plan, in which more and more patients are admitted to the study until a difference is proved to exist. For this method, a maximum number of cases is often stated (Armitage
  1975; Bross 1952; McPherson 1977).

With sequential plans, usually less patients are
needed than with preset ones. However, there are
situations in which the sequential method should
be decided against. Wherever the observation period
is very much longer than the recruitment period,
sequential plans have no advantage. Moreover, ad-

ministrative considerations often necessitate knowing exactly in advance how much time a study must
take (e.g., multicentre studies).

In designing a study, one may choose a "mixed" plan
(neither purely sequential nor the opposite): after
a pre-determined number of cases is reached, it is
decided upon whether the experiment is continued
or not. Figures on numbers of cases are found in
MEYDRICH and KUPPER (1978), and in SCHLESSELMAN
(1974).

Selection
of patients   The study protocol must contain definitions of the
inclusion and exclusion criteria for the subjects.
The following factors, among others, should be duly
considered (BURLEY 1976; EDERER 1975; JOHNSON, JOHN-
SON 1977):
- age
- sex
- type and severity of illnesses
- previous and present therapy
Reasons for exclusion are, as a rule:
- pregnancy
- critical illness
- refusal to participate
If the restrictions due to the above factors are
severe and the number of exclusion criteria is
large, the number of patients available for the
study may be too small. Otherwise, there may be
some undesirable selection.

The criteria established for inclusion and exclusion must remain the same during the entire course
of the study. No patient classified as eligible by
the said criteria may be excluded from participation.

Efficacy
criteria   The choice and the number of efficacy criteria result from the problem as formulated. For evaluation
of therapeutic success, only few outcome variables
should be used, if this is possible. Such variables

may be symptoms of the disease to be treated as planned, survival time or the duration of the remission achieved. If too many efficacy criteria are chosen, difficulties ensue with regard to predetermination of the number of cases required and to the interpretation of the results of multivariate statistical tests (Jesdinsky 1978; Johnson, Johnson 1977).

Interference, influencing and concomitant variables

The restriction on the number of outcome variables does not preclude that a considerable number of variables is documented during a therapeutic study to eliminate interference variables on the one hand and to generate new hypotheses on the other (Johnson, Johnson 1999; Meier 1975). Interference variables cannot be adequately taken into account during the design stage, but may be documented for retrospective processing in the statistical analysis. Interference variables are, for example, secondary diagnoses or riks factors. Influencing variables (or parameters) are such factors as the primary diagnosis, the therapy, the age of the patient, etc., and must be taken into consideration in the experimental design. Concomitant variables are additional ones documented, e.g., for the purpose of generating new hypotheses.

Study types

The different study types and the indications therefore have already been discussed. Some important study types are recalled in the following:
- controlled clinical trial (prospective and randomized)
- intervention study (prospective and experimental)
- case-control study (retrospective)
- observational study (non-randomized)
- register

Most of these types of studies may be open or blind, monocentric or multicentric (Jesdinsky, 1979; Johnson, Johnson 1977; Maxwell 1968).

Dosage plans

If it is established that a fixed and constant

dose of a therapeutic drug is effective and non-
toxic despite individual variations, a trial may
be conducted using this dosage. The necessity of
individually tailored dosage often encountered in
clinical practice must be taken into account in
the design stage of a therapeutic study. The planning and the implementation of a study become more
complicated in such cases, but the ensuing results
are medically more realistic. The dose needed to
attain a given effect may even become the main criterion on which a study is judged (Bruley 1976;
Johnson, Johnson 1977; World Health Organization
1975).

Examination dates and the time of measurement	Dates of examinations and the exact time of each measurement must be recorded (study protocol). In course-oriented studies, it is a rule to establish fixed intervals between such examinations and measurements. However, in event-oriented studies, such times depend on the taking place of one or more events, such as a change in the clinical picture, side-effects, etc. (Johnson, Johnson 1977).
Methods of evaluation	These, including planned statistical tests, are to be defined in the study protocol in their connection with all other aspects of the design of the trial in question (Jesdinsky 1978; Johnson, Johnson 1977).

2.2. Documentation

Reliable and complete documentation is an indispensable condition for
any and every scientific presentation of facts. The best experimental
design, the most suitable analysis and the utmost thoroughness in data
processing are worthless without proper documentation of each case and
of the entire study.

Describing and establishing the documentation	It is not possible to describe in generalized terms which details are to be documented. This depends on the problem at hand, the situation, the design of the trial, the available resources, and many other

factors. Too voluminous documentation are usually badly and incompletely followed; however, the facts relevant to the said problem may, on the other hand, not be omitted. The forms used and the instructions for their use must be previously spelled out in detail, so that there is no ambiguity involved in filling them in. The questionnaire and, as complete as possible, a description of the documentation of cases are important parts of the study protocol and must be given in full detail. The evidential potential of a study may, in most cases, be appraised by a scrutiny of the above-mentioned documents (Köpcke, Überla 1978; World Health Organization 1975).

Uniformity

The forms used in collecting data for the documentation of the cases must be standardized for all cases and control groups, and be used uniformly in all instances; this precaution must be taken to ensure the best possible approximation to observational equality. If different forms are used to document the same facts for the same subjects, serious differences may be introduced into the data via the forms. Hence, observational equality requires uniform documentation forms for all subjects. This is what is called acquisitional equality which may not be violated in the process of documentation (Köpcke, Überla 1978).

Completeness

Documentation must be presented for each case, even if subjects drop out or show unfavourable results. The completeness of the documentation is a matter of scientific honesty, as selection of the "favourable" instances may furnish any result desired. This means that all subjects admitted to the study must be completely documented. The questionnaires and the other documents must be filled in without any data being omitted. Any missing data interfere in an uncontrollable way with the result of the comparison intended (Köpcke, Überla 1978).

Usefullness and effectiveness	The questionnaire should be designed in such a way that filling it in is as easy as possible. Hence, the process of examination should be followed in its temporal sequence. Good documentation takes up not much more time than that needed for the actual examinations. All papers involved should be designed in such a way as to establish whether, how and/or how much data are to be read automatically. The purpose of the forms is, besides that of supporting those filling them in, also to effectively generate automatically readable data documents. These two objectives are often incompatible and must be weighed against each other in such cases (Grady 1976; Köpcke, Überla 1978).
Logical and systems aspects	A form used for documentation should be logically structured and/or conform to an appropriate system. The form should follow the course of the examination(s), bring laboratory findings into sufficient contrast to others, reflect the time sequence of the data acquisition and make important information, e.g., outcome variables, stand out clearly. The system used - and embodied by headings, colours, separate blocks, special forms, etc. - should not be too detailed, as this may cause problems. However, this system should be recognizable both for the persons filling in the forms and the ones charged with evaluating them. Documentation papers with unrecognizable structure and haphazardly scattered variables are more difficult to fill in, are penalized by a relatively high error ratio and also "document" insufficient preparation for the clinical trial in question (Grady 1976; Köpcke, Überla 1978).
Types of variables	Each clinical observation is made on an observational unit with respect to a definite "feature" or variable. Such units are usually the subjects, but also may be case histories or ECG curves recorded at a given time. An observational unit is the smallest unit for statistically oriented experi-

ments or statistical analysis. Such units must be
carefully defined before the study is begun: this
is an obvious condition for meaningful evaluation.
It is especially important to know whether a given
subject occurs once or more than once in a study
(if once, the observational unit is this subject;
otherwise, it is his "case").

For each observational unit, a documentation sheet
for the observed features of this unit is filled
in. Features may be qualitative or quantitative;
the latter are either continuous or discrete
(Johnson, Johnson 1977; Proppe 1975).

Qualitative
variables

A feature (i.e., a variable) is called qualitative,
if it is expressed in categories or classes that
are not distinguished numerically but conceptually.
Examples for such variables are: sex, death/survi-
val, drop-out (as against the opposite), occupation and diagnosis. Arbitrary numbers may be assigned to the possible "values" of qualitative
variables, as in "male = 1, female = 2". This procedure is called coding. Determining the proper
code is an important and timeconsuming task involved in the documentation of any clinical trial
(Immich 1975; Köpcke, Überla 1978).

Quantitative
variables

A variable is called quantitative if its values
can be numerically expressed in a way allowing
comparisons of greater to smaller numbers. Examples
are: marks achieved in school, single vs. multiple
positives, weight, height, number of children, blood
pressure, results of laboratory tests, etc.. Quantitative variables are either discrete or continuous.
The latter can assume all values within a given
range (e.g., height, weight, blood pressure and
most of the laboratory variables). Discrete variables, which are usually the result of counting,
can only have a limited number of definite values
(e.g., the number of siblings). Continuous variables usually result from measurement (Köpcke,
Überla 1978).

Hard and soft data	This differentiation is verbal and more or less arbitrary, and is not very important in documentation. Laboratory and other measurements, which are regarded as "hard" data by doctors, are frequently "softer" than data from questionnaires or psychological tests, as far as validity and reliability are concerned. We must avoid, as far as possible, the use of concepts which may be modified by subjective impressions of an observer. Each documentation sheet must provide adequate space for remarks in free text, in order to record observers' impressions and unforeseen events (if any). The amount of space to be allotted to this purpose depends on the objectives of the study. Such free text can, as a rule, be coded only roughly (and even this presents difficulties), and is hard to evaluate in quantitative terms. Free text is out of the question for outcome variables. However, such text does furnish useful qualitative information and is a suitable supplement to the main body of data, as it motivates the observers and gives them full freedom to express their observations (Köpcke, Überla 1978).
Development of documentation forms	Development of such forms requires that the above-mentioned relevant points are taken into due consideration. After the problem is formulated and a rough outline of the study exists (as to subjects, outcome variables and experimental design), the variables to be raised for documentation are identified: scrutiny of the pertinent literature and conferences with colleagues are required to find the most suitable parameters for the facts on which the research is to be done. A first draft of the documentation plan is then discussed; this requires examining each variable in detail as to type, possible values, and aspects bearing on form-filling, coding and usefulness. Automatically readable data-bearing documents are to be defined and the structure of the documentation sheet including the underlying system must be decided upon; the effectiveness, suitability and user ease involved

must be reviewed in detail. In most cases, several drafts are needed at this stage. The last draft is used for a trial run, for which a small number of cases is fully documented. The planned evaluation must be tailored to the documentation sheet. The final edition and the printing of the forms, which are binding for the entire study, complete this development phase (Bennet, Ritchie 1975; Berche, Anderson 1974; Grady 1976).

The form and detail of the data-acquisition documents (questionnaires, etc.) depends on a decision on how the documented facts are to be read into a data-processing unit. There are, in principle, four media to choose from: punch cards - perforated tapes - magnetic discettes, documents for marking, forms for document readers and on-line data collection systems.

Punch cards /
perforated tapes/
magnetic discettes

When cards (or tapes) are being punched, it must be arranged for that the person charged with punching the documented data does so in the same columns of the cards for the same, pre-established types of data. This implies giving each variable fixed, numbered columns. In many cases, it is useful to include a section for this purpose (the "punching section") on the right margin of the documentation form. The filled-in form must be supplemented by coding the data it contains, and entering this coded material in the punching section. The punching itself may then follow as the third phase of the acquisition process. This allows freedom in designing the form, which in turn makes for exactness and freedom in filling it in. However, it must be noted that the entire body of data must be processed three times. Alternatively, one may include the information needed for punching in the form itself; however, the form is usually rendered more complicated by so doing. This may be tolerated by experienced personnel, but may cause some confusion among doctors. The advantage of this method is telescoping three stages of activity into two.

A third variation consists in using a carbon copy:
the leading page contains the form without a punching section, and the carbon copy only the latter.
This also makes for freedom of design of the form
and two-stage processing, and provides a separate
document for the punchers. However, the work needed
for development takes more time, and the carbon
copies that must be provided make for additional
cost (Köhler 1975; Köpcke, Überla 1978).

Documents for marking

Such documents (slips) are used in that the appropriate answers are marked (e.g., underlined) with
a soft pencil for automatic reading; hence, no
punching is needed. The prerequisite to this is,
however, that the possible values of all variables
are established before the study is begun. Quantitative variables are difficult to cover in this
way and may be subject to additional errors when
treated in this manner. Hence, many quantitative
variables do not qualify for this kind of processing. A further handicap consists in the relatively
expensive training of the personnel charged with
the marking activity, as relatively small errors
in marking may lead to false values being read. To
sum up: the method is useful in studies involving
a great amount of data; with trials involving a
few hundred subjects, it should be chosen only in
exceptional cases (Köhler 1975; Köpcke, Überla
1978).

Document-reader forms

Document reader can process certain types of cha-
racters from special typewriters without any pre-
processing being needed. This is important in cases
involving extensive free-text input and a large
number of cases; however, this advantage is confined, in the field of clinical studies, to exceptional projects involving unusual numbers of subjects. There are modern document-reading machines
capable of reading hand-written numbers; if these
are to be utilized, the development of appropriate
forms is costly, special paper is needed and train-

ing personnel requires great care. Hence, forms for document readers are useful only for large-scale studies or for data of the same type that are acquired in the same manner during a series of studies (Köhler 1975; Köpcke, Überla 1978).

On-line data collection systems

Nowadays data collection is often performed directly on-line at a terminal. With the modern data-bank systems like SIR (Robinson 1980) marks with explaining texts are generated which makes data collection more easier. At the same time a first error checking is done by the data-bank system so that errors can easily and directly be corrected by the user.

2.3. Organization

Therapeutic studies are complex systems with very detailed objectives. Hence, they usually require concerted action by a number of specialists. Frequently, a number of clinics must be jointly managed - with respect to the study - for an extended period of time; such management becomes the more difficult, the larger the study and the number of participants is. Therefore, the organizational problem should not be underrated with regard to the implementation of therapeutic studies.

Responsibilities

The responsible planning group for a therapeutic study should consist of clinicians, methodologists, and experts for the therapy to be assessed; this group should be listed by individual names in the study plan (Jesdinsky 1978; Nicholson 1976).

A doctor should be the head of the study group and bear the overall responsibility for the design and implementation of the study, without thereby restricting the personal responsibility of the doctors involved for the patients under their care. In multicentre studies, a doctor in charge is needed for each individual centre. As a rule, a Study Secretary will be needed for multicentre projects for purposes of coordination and also to free the head of the study group from administrative and organizational tasks.

A methodologist (e.g., a statistician) shares the responsibility with the head of the study group for experimental design, design of documentation forms, data processing and statistical analysis. According to the type of study planned, others must bear the responsibility for certain centralized tasks (pathology, laboratory, etc.).

Institutions

With multicentric studies, the question of the type and number of the institutions involved must be answered during the planning stage. The study plan must contain the inclusion and exclusion criteria for the participation of individual clinics. One of the most important parameters in this regard is the number of subjects each clinic can contribute to the study. Other criteria for selection of clinics are equipment and personnel and techniques of observation and treatment. A centre for documentation, data processing and statistics must be consulted for the following: planning of experiments, design of documentation forms, review and supervision of documentation, ongoing preparation of statistics, statistical analysis, and the entire area of data processing. Further centralized tasks may, in some cases, need appropriate centres to which work is referred (Selbmann 1978; Snell 1976).

Personnel

Details on number and qualifications of the personnel needed belong to the essentials of the study plan (Johnson, Johnson 1977; Snell 1976). This holds true not only for doctors and scientists, but equally for personnel required in administrative and technical capacities. It must be made clear which personnel must be recruited for which tasks, and which activities are to be performed by existing personnel. The period of occupation according to the time schedule must be set out for each participant. Personnel plans are to be drawn up separately for the planning group, the project management and coordination and central services (statistics, evaluation, laboratory, pathology, etc.).

Finances   It must be clarified which funds are needed by
                  which participating institutions, and for which
                  reasons. The following areas must be differentiated
                  (Nicholson 1976; Sondik et al. 1974):
                  - cost of central services (such as the study bu-
                    reau, coordination meetings, travel, paper and
                    printing, statistics and evaluation, laboratory
                    and pathology), and
                  - expenses incurred by participating clinics, such
                    as infrastructure (equipment and personnel, in-
                    dependent of the number of patients) and expen-
                    ses on the number of patients (for treatment,
                    documentation, etc.).
                  The cost of work delegated to third parties is
                  deemed to constitute an integral part of the "cost
                  of central services".

                  In addition to the foregoing, the expenses should
                  be itemized according to the following headings:
                  - personnel expenses, including details on quali-
                    fications, duties, and scope of work of each
                    worker
                  - a list of instruments and other equipment used,
                    with cost estimation
                  - travel expenses, separately listed as to domestic
                    and abroad
                  - material used up
                  - computing costs
                  - rent
                  - contracts with third parties
                  - other expenses

Time   The time needed for the different stages according
schedule   to plan must be stated; a "milestone plan" estab-
                  lishes the important fixed points of a therapeutic
                  study. The proper timing of each part of the study
                  must be continuously monitored in order to find
                  out organizational faults such as non-adherence to
                  the time schedule for observations and other devia-
                  tions from the time schedule laid down in the mile-
                  stone plan, and to correct such faults while there
                  is still time to do so (George, Desu 1974; Jesdinsky
                  1978; Johnson, Johnson 1977).

It is especially important to terminate a therapeutic study within the period planned for the
project. The coordinator is responsible for ensuring such cooperation of all centres involved that
the study may be terminated as soon as possible.
The study protocol should contain criteria enabling the head of the study group to exclude at
any time such centres which do not cooperate in
the proper way.

Supervision of judgemental activity

It must be ensured that all cases are judged according to unambiguously defined criteria. This is
only possible if a meticulously kept study protocol is supplemented by continuous supervision.
How the latter is put into practice depends on
both the type and the size of a therapeutic study.
Independent assessment of admission criteria, therapeutic success, laboratory measurements, etc.
by a group of non-participating experts is hardly
possible except for large-scale monocentre studies
or multicentre ones (Selbmann 1978).

Ethical and legal supervision

Each therapeutic study must take place within the
bounds of generally recognized ethical and legal
standards (van Eimeren, Überla 1975; Hasskarl
1978; Hasskarl, Kleinsorge 1979; Meier 1975; Revidierte Deklaration von Helsinki 1975; Smith 1977;
Staak, Weiser 1978; Tancredi 1975). Such standards
imply (Lewandowski 1979):
- acceptable experimental risk
- experienced leadership and qualified personnel
- pharmacological and toxicological tests
- patients insurance.

The informed consent of the patients with respect
to the following aspects is indispensable (Berger,
Stallones 1977):
- explanation of the study and of the reasons for
  undertaking it
- information on possible risks and side-effects
- information on possible advantages

- statement that no better alternative therapies
  are available
- readiness to answer every question of a patient
- notification that any patient may terminate his
  participation in the study at any time.

An independent group not charged with caring for
study patients should continuously supervise the
action and guarantee adherence to the rules, especially concerning informed consent of the patients before agreeing to take part in the study.
According to MAY (1975), this group should include
not only doctors, but also lawyers, statisticians
and representatives of the nursing personnel.

Quality
control

The specific methods of examinations used in a
study should be subjected to quality control. This
holds true not only for the laboratory methods,
the most of which are checked routinely by means
of standard quality control experiments. Variables
which may be influenced by subjective factors must
be carefully checked as to their observational variability, especially if such variables are exclusion or inclusion criteria (e.g., histological
diagnoses from biopsies). Checking is also required
for the documentation, especially regarding the
reliability and exactness of the data entered in
the sheets (Breslow 1978; Ederer 1975; Gordis 1979;
Jesdinsky 1978).

Comparability
in multicentre
studies

In such studies, measurements which are criteria
for in- or exclusion or for stratification should
be made at a single centre (e.g., by central laboratories, central randomization, and central expert groups). This is the only way to minimize the
differences between the participating clinics. Com-
parable conditions with regard to these clinics
may be created by standardizing the equipment and
personnel, the organization, and techniques of observation, treatment and assessment of outcome
(Selbmann 1978).

Unexpected	Unexpected discoveries either made with the pa-
discoveries	tients treated within the scope of the study or
and termination	in the literature may never lead to introduction
of treatment	of new problem formulations while a therapeutic

Unexpected discoveries either made with the patients treated within the scope of the study or in the literature may never lead to introduction of new problem formulations while a therapeutic study is in process; such discoveries may, however, be a reason for planning a new study or terminating the current one (Breslow 1978; Bulpitt 1975).

If the treatment of a patient is terminated, the reason therefore must be documented in full detail. The study protocol should, however, contain a list for foreseeable reasons for such termination, such as (Jesdinsky 1978):
- Revoking of consent to the therapy by the patient
- Removal of the patient from the study on medical grounds, such as side-effects, failure of the treatment or new illnesses leading to such removal
- "technical" reasons, such as transferral to another ward or non-confirmation of the originally suspected diagnosis.

Publication of the study

Before a therapeutic study is begun, it must be agreed on in which manner the results of the study will be published. In this regard, the important questions of authorship (joint/and/or individual publications), the channels used (technical report(s), a book, articles in journals and/or papers read at symposia) and prospective readers (clinicians, methodologists, politicians, etc.) must be settled. Practical suggestions for publications may be found in HAWKINS (1976); methodological aspects are discussed in O'FALLON et al. (1978).

2.4. Statistical analysis

The planning for therapeutic studies is not confined only to the design of the experimental process, the establishing of secondary conditions and the definition of procedures of implementation: a most important part of the necessary preparation is the planning for adequate analysis and evaluation of the results obtained from the entire research effort (Selbmann 1978).

Pre-processing of the data	We know from experience that more findings result from data collection in therapeutic studies that one can evaluate in the available time and use for the final report. For the best possible utilization of this entire body of information, we recommend pre-processing the data in such a way that they can be made available to other researchers (with due regard to data protection) for their future work. Pre-processing includes coding of qualitative data (such as diagnosis, occupation, etc.) and is completed when all the data are stored in automatically readable form on punched cards, magnetic tape, magnetic disks and similiar media (Immich 1975; Jesdinsky 1978; Köhler 1975; Proppe 1975).
Data read-in	It must be known before the beginning of a therapeutic study which type of computing facility is available for analysis. The details of data storage and read-in must be agreed upon with the statistician and/or the head of the computing centre, according to the technical status of this centre (Köhler 1975a/b).
Plausibility and error checking	The opportunity of fast and reliable handling of large quantities of data by means of a computer is an advantage only if the quality of the data themselves can be relied on. Hence, the checking of clinical data is an important and indispensable task preceding the analysis of therapeutic studies. Whereas mistakes as to facts may be checked only with great labour and expense (or, at worst, not at all), the data may be checked as to formal errors far more thoroughly and speedily with computer aid than by conventional methods; this is an area in which electronic data processing comes to the fore. Checking for formal errors includes the following:

- checking for completeness of the data
- checking for impossible codes
- checking for permissible ranges of values
- checking for incompatibilities of all kinds.
It should be attempted to correct all the data
shown by the checking process to be in error, as
far as this is possible (Wagner 1975).

Another way of checking the quality of the data
is effecting plausibility checks for bodies of
data (e.g., end-figure analysis). If these aggre-
gates are large enough, one may postulate even
distribution without knowing whether the individual values are correct. Quantity and quality of
deviations allow deductions as to the size and
possible source of the errors to be made. However,
correction of individual data is not possible by
this method.

Programs
for analysis

As of now, a considerable number of computer programs exist for statistical analysis of medical
data. The most widely used program systems are
known as SAS (SAS 1981), BMDP (Dixon 1981), and
SPSS (Bentel et al. 1980). In recent years, program systems for interactive analysis, like SIR
(Robinson 1980) have appeared. We recommend using
such existing programs if they are kmown to be free
of errors, meet the technical requirements of the
user, and have acceptable input and, above all, out-
put facilities. The expense in terms of time and
money involved in using such programs with different
computers for the analysis of statistical variables
should not be underrated. In each individual case,
the expert in charge of the analysis should consider
whether a program of his own may be more economical.

Description

The analysis of therapeutic studies consists of a
descriptive and a deductive part. Descriptive analyses allows one to obtain lucid and speedy information on the results of the experiments, but may
be misleading in that scale manipulations or trans-
formations produce false impressions. Descriptive
statistics may be presented as frequency tables,

histograms, graphs, and as data on means, scatter, correlation, regression, etc. (Ambler 1977; Koller 1975).

Statistical
tests

A statistical test is used to obtain an answer to the question whether a given therapy produces an effect differing to that of the therapy of the control groups. All statistical tests are designed to generalize results of observations in that they enable inferences to be made from observed samples to an underlying population (Ambler 1977; Jesdinsky 1979; Selbmann 1978). Every statistical test results in one of the following two statements :
- the therapy groups differ more than can be expected from chance, i.e., one may assume with an error probability less than 1% or 5% that the therapies have differing effects;
- one must continue to assume that the effect of the therapies is essentially equal, as a difference cannot be shown to exist.

For meaningful application of statistical tests, specific conditions must be fulfilled such as special distributions and/or a minimum number of cases, or specified procedures. It is the responsibility of the statistician in charge to arrange for these conditions being fulfilled (if possible, during the design stage of the project), to obtain a correct application of each test in the subsequent analysis.

2.5. Evaluation of the Study

The final report on a therapeutic study should contain not only statistical analysis and interpretation of the facts, but also a detailed analysis of the design, documentation and organization of the project (Levy 1977).

Design
analysis

This is required to elucidate whether randomization, stratification and patient selection were implemented according to the pre-existing design, and to find out to what extent this procedure has produced structural equality of the groups compared.

Examination of the documentation

This inquiry is a quality check as to fulfilment of the requirements (uniformity, completeness, suitability, and logical and systematic criteria). If the study protocol was modified during the study period, the reasons for and the effects of so doing must be stated.

Observational equality

Especially where a multicentre study is involved, it must be ascertained whether standardization of observational and therapeutic techniques and of judgmental criteria has resulted in the observational equality required for the study.

Personnel

It should be ascertained whether the personnel requirements set out in the original plan - for administrative, medical, scientific and technical positions - was realistic. It should be determined when and where more or less personnel than planned for were needed. Furthermore, reasons for temporary or total vacancies should be analyzed and the performance of the workers in each area reviewed.

Operating expenses

Proper accounting for the materials used up in a study is an obvious requirement. Besides this, all areas should be reviewed in which the original budget was not or could not be adhered to; the results may have a bearing on future studies, and recommendations should be made if this is seen to be reasonable.

Cooperation

The cooperation between the institutions and between the people involved should be reviewed; if there are shortcomings in this respect, the reason for this should be sought out and set out.

Legal and ethical problems

Legal and ethical problems encountered in the course of the study (such as unexpected side-effects, or discoveries that jeopardized the study) should be described, and the action taken on account of such problems set out and explained.

Time schedule	Evaluation of the study includes answering the question whether the time schedule for the project was realistic regarding its stages (design, initiation, treatment and observation of the patients, analysis).
Statistics	With regard to the statistical analysis, it must be clarified whether the conditions for the application of all statistical methods used were fulfilled, and whether the test involved were correctly executed.
Interpretation	Interpretation, including generalization, of the results of a therapeutic study should be carefully weighed and not exceed the limits set by the observations made. Such interpretation depends on the analysis of all factors which could possibly have affected the results. We must expressly warn the reader not to make the statistical significance or non-significance of differences in critical variables the equivalent of a medical recommendation or condemnation of a therapeutic method. The size and medical relevance of such differences should be much more of a criterion for such action than mere statistical significance. Moreover, the results of an individual study should be judged in their relationship to the results of other studies on the same problem (Jesdinsky 1978).
Effects of a study and conclusions	Besides the evaluation criteria based on the study and its results, there are also "external" criteria leading to an opinion on a therapeutic study. Its success may be evidenced by changes in therapeutic reality. The opinion of the scientific community (voiced in criticism, quotations and general discussion) is important. Finally, it should be asked whether the therapy in question has changed hitherto existing knowledge and/or given rise to new ideas and concepts.

3. Special Problems in the Organization and Implementation of Multicentre Therapeutic Studies

This chapter is a supplement to the checklist as to a number of points that lead to difficulties with multicentre studies. Experience with such studies has shown that much effort is required to solve these problems.

3.1. Prerequisites to Successful Cooperative Research

Cooperative versus individual research

Multicentre studies require specific behavior and attitudes from the contributing scientists and doctors. The individual is a member of a research group formed to reach a common goal. Prerequisites to successful cooperative research are leanings toward cooperation, agreement, creativity and innovation within a group and de-emphasizing of individual interests in favour of a common cause. This includes adapting oneself to a research situation differing in a number of points from individual research. In studies carried out in a single place by individual researchers or by a small team under a leading investigator, the innovative and creative powers and the experience and scientific interests of individuals come to the fore, and there is usually great flexibility as to procedure. There are no special problems connected with standardization of data acquisition and monitoring of the situation in which this is done. The individual-research situation is characterized by its transparency and by minimal pressure toward agreement in addition to rapid feedback enabling one to assess a current study from results obtained and to make changes in the project whenever this is needed.

This degree of flexibility does not exist in cooperative projects. After the study protocol has been established by the participants and the study proper has begun, strict adherence to this document is binding on all involved. If changes are deemed necessary in the course of the study, they

must, again, be agreed on. Such measures depend
not on the results obtained in a single clinic,
but on those found in all participating clinics.
This alone prevents short-term adjustments to
current results. As a rule, central data monitoring is performed rather infrequently (one to three
times a year); the outcome of this may lead to decisions on continuation or termination of the
study and/or changes in the study protocol (Hagans
1974).

**Requirements
for successful
planning and
implementation
of therapeutic
studies**

All experts should have a share in the planning of
a multicentre study who play an important part in
the subsequent implementation. At this stage,
close cooperation between doctors and methodologists is a matter of great consequence. The detailed formulation of the study protocol requires
a number of common sessions and group discussions,
for which sufficient time should be provided.
There is often a tendency to begin with a study
before all the details have become clear. A draft
of the study protocol should be submitted to an
independent group of experts (such as a review
committee) for examination, so as to detect and
correct errors and/or omissions without delay.

Before patients are admitted to the study, all
doctors and other personnel involved in the implementation but not in the planning must be informed
in detail on the procedures to be followed. These
are concerned with patient selection, administration of therapy, required examinations and observations, and the filling in of the documentation
sheets. If more than five clinics participate in
the study, it is advisable to entrust only a few of
the doctors responsible for the study in the different clinics with the central direction of the project. At this time, the necessary central facilities must already exist, such as laboratories,
pathology services, dosimetry and regular data
quality control, and data analysis and evaluation.

In multicentre studies, arrangements must be made
for interim presentations of results from time to
time, so that the further course of the study may
be decided on according to the information thus
received. Decisions on changes of the study protocol should be made by a group of experts not involved in administering the treatments. Successful
cooperative studies are wound up by the publication
of the results, for which task a group should be
chosen from the participants (the "writing committee").

Cooperation with practising doctors	Multicentre studies often require cooperation with practising physicians (Bundesärztekammer 1978). Past experience with studies on heart and circula- tory diseases show that participation of practising doctors leads to problems concerning adherence to the study protocol and data quality control. It is often not ensured that the therapy is conducted according to plan and that complications are repor- ted to the clinic conducting the study. Here, both doctor and patient compliance and their control are a significant and partly unsolved problem (Agras, Marshall 1979).
"Quorum" of participating clinics	The participation of clinics in multicentre studies should entail specific requirements. Among these is a stipulated minimum number of patients per year admitted to the study. Such conditions for partici- pation exist with the European Organization for Re- search and Treatment of Cancer. However, such "quo- rum" requirements should include quality criteria as to the clinic and the physicians participating in a study. Implementation of such studies and the intensity of care for the patients involved require material and manpower resources in addition to spe- cific experience.

3.2. Quality Control

Especially in multicentre studies, it must be made sure that the study protocol is adhered to and that the study is conducted according to this protocol. Quality control includes both external checking of the participating clinics by the coordinating centre, and checks within individual clinics. Both is done to control observational errors.

Comprehensive quality control often meets with resistance on the part of the physicians participating in a study, especially if the measures taken are felt to be unreasonable and/or disruptive. Such problems may be avoided if the purpose of all measures involved in quality control are discussed at the outset, and the participating doctors in the clinics are convinced that its purpose is not supervision of their action but the providing of aids for successful implementation of the study. Hence, the objective of comprehensive quality control should not only be seen to consist of the uncovering of errors, but also to lie in a common quest for solutions.

Cost-benefit aspects are also decisive for the extent of quality control. Too much quality control is just as wrong as too little. However, a minimum of quality control is always needed; otherwise, one may well feel safe without this being reflected in the facts. WILLIAMS has characterized such situations by remarking, "The only way to be comfortable about data and inference quality is never to check" (Williams 1979, p. 702).

Aspects of a comprehensive quality control programme	Simultaneously with the "strategic" schedule for planning and implementation of the study, a comprehensive quality control programme should be prepared for the study: this should cover all aspects of the study and its progress in time, such as responsibilities, study documents, data, publications, etc., and should not be confined to data quality control only (Williams 1979).
Responsibility and Competence	Quality control includes, among other aspects, providing for scientific responsibility and competence for the study. A two level committee may be recommended, viz.,

- the coordinating centre consisting of a limited number of scientists participating in the study, and of external experts
- representatives of all clinics, hospitals and

other institutions participating in the study.

The responsibilities and competences involved in implementing a study must be stipulated in detail. This concerns the parts played by the coordinating centre, the sponsoring institution and the clinics, and all activities for communications and the exchange of views. This latter area includes organizing and conducting conferences and meetings on the status of the study, special aspects, and the research done in individual clinics participating in the study, in addition to preparing regular reports on results obtained.

Study
documents

The most important study document is the protocol. This must be supplemented by instructions covering details of procedure. Both the protocol and the instructions should be written in such a way that not only participants in the study but also others are able to become fully informed as to the purpose, the context and the course of the study. It must be ensured that the protocol and the instructions are read by all concerned, and that current versions are used. Moreover, care should be taken to keep the instructions intelligible, accurate and easy to follow. Graphs and diagrams may add clarity to the instructions and help to avoid problems in their application.

The design of questionnaires and other forms for documentation requires special care. Efforts must be made toward user ease and unambiguous instructions as to handling the forms. A trial run with real users should be made. Furthermore, it must be established what is done if forms are lost, who receives the original forms and how errors in documentation should be corrected. For the latter, it is necessary to be able to find out from individual forms who had acquired and documented the data.

The pilot stage	Each large study should, if possible, begin with a pilot stage; its purpose is to test the theoretically planned course of the study as to feasibility in a real situation and to make corrections where needed. Before the study is begun, all direct participants require instruction. This is best done by the group charged with checking the data acquisition, i.e., the coordinating centre.
Data quality control	By data quality control, it is intended to achieve reproducibility of results obtained, given the same conditions. Such reproducibility or reliability of the data may be endangered by observational errors, especially by systematic errors leading to bias. An important method of eliminating such errors is the "blind" technique, which should be used wherever this is feasible and necessary and be checked as to being strictly followed. A realibility check may be confined to samples of patients for which examinations are repeated, and/or documents are "blindly" evaluated by a third party.
	Quality control is expensive in terms of time and money. Hence, the amount of checking done should be reasonably related to the importance of the data in question. However, quality control should never be restricted only to checking adherence to inclusion and exclusion criteria, but also include data storage, all methods of measurement and calculation, and also coding and data transfer.
Reporting	A quality control programme must also cover the writing of interim reports and of the final report on a study. Regarding this, it must be checked whether an appropriate statistical analysis of the data was performed and whether the computations involved were both error-free and correctly applied. It is most important to choose the proper words and phrases for the text of the report, so that ambiguity and false understanding of the results are avoided.

External quality control by the coordinating centre	This is continual feedback (on details of adherence to the study protocol in the individual clinics) to the coordinating centre and its data processing staff. The purpose of this activity is - maintaining open communication channels between the coordinating centre and the participating clinics - ensuring clarity as to responsibility and competences in the clinics - uniformity of procedure in the different clinics - monitoring of the data raised in these clinics. According to experience gathered in the "Lipid Research Clinics Programme", regular telephone calls and visits to the clinics in addition to constant error-checking of all data in the data processing centre are the methods best suited for such external quality control (Mowery, Williams 1979).
Regular telephone conversation with the clinician responsible for the study	Telephone calls are the simplest method of regular contact with the participating clinics. Such conversations should take place once a week or at least once a fortnight. In such talks between a member of the coordinating centre and the responsible clinician, a number of questions may be handled, such as : - errors in the forms forwarded to the data processing centre - training of new personnel - current status of the study - problems created by personnel turnover and/or non-availability of equipment needed for purposes of the study - problems concerning handling of study documents, etc.. Such telephone exchanges are, of course, useful only if it is ensured that important information is properly forwarded and that the necessary action is taken.

Regular
visits to
clinics

Members of the coordinating centre should visit
the participating clinics at regular intervals.
Such visits allow direct exchange of information
in official meetings and during informal talks
with participating physicians and other health
personnel. In the joint meetings, problems involved in fulfilling the study protocol should be
the prime topic discussed. These include all questions arising from changes in the protocol, whether
past or planned. The visit allows, in addition,
opportunity for direct observation and for taking
part in all study activities such as medical examinations and data acquisition. The members of
the coordinating centre thus obtain important
insight into difficulties posed by the study protocol. The outcome of each visit to a clinic
should be described in writing and be sent to the
chairman of the coordinating centre, the head of
the clinic visited and, if applicable, to the
sponsoring organization.

Quality control
of incoming
data in the
data processing
centre

The data processing centre should perform, besides
its current data quality controls, periodic data
checks with respect to the clinics. The documents
from each clinic should be regularly reviewed as
to :
- completeness and readability of entries and adherence to the protocol
- systematic observational errors.
The results should be reported to the clinics; the
coordinating centre should confer with clinics
evidencing problems on solutions enabling future
avoidance of the errors in question.

Problems of
internal
quality
control

Monitoring the situations in which the medical
examinations etc. are performed in the participating clinics is called internal quality control.
EVANS (1979) has found that this is, as a rule,
the weakest part of overall data quality control,
as clinicians are understandably more interested
in the result of their work than in asking them-

selves whether the data they acquire meet certain
requirements as to quality. Moreover, 'the aim of
medical training is the availability of good physicians, not of clinical research workers. Besides
many doctors hardly know that observation and
acquisition of data may give rise to a multitude
of errors without ignorance or carelessness being
involved. There is also very often a failure to
correctly estimate the amount of work which can
be done in a given period of time. Whenever physicians participate in studies, they should know
that they are prone to observational errors and
cannot do everything themselves; they should, moreover, know that standardized procedure based on
the study protocol is required for checking for
observational errors and to allow them to delegate
routine tasks to others. The importance of such
standardized procedure is borne out by a study carried out by the Roswell Park Memorial Institute,
according to which systematic patient care based
on a protocol enhanced the quality of such care
and of the data acquired more than having the
patients treated by one and the same physician
(Grimm et al. 1975).

Informing participating clinicians on the purpose of the study	Clinicians are a team which works best if it is fully conversant with the purpose of the study. The doctors examining the patients should know the problems at the root of the study, the steps involved in its implementation, inclusion and exclusion criteria, methods of treatment and their ramifications and the rules stipulated in the study protocol for data acquisition and documentation. The principle investigator in an individual clinic should make sure that this knowledge really exists.
Supervision of study activities by the principle investigator	The most important task of this physician with respect to internal quality control is to arrange for the study protocol to be followed and to prevent occurrence of observational errors. As to the former, problems may be expected regarding in-

clusion criteria, call-up of patients in long-term follow-up programmes, termination of treatment on account of side-effects, proper formulation of results of therapy, etc.. The principle investigator should keep himself informed on the quality of the data acquisition by participating in examinations performed by the doctors administering the therapy and by repeating such examinations himself from time to time.

Avoidance of patient drop-out

Such drop-out may become a serious problem, especially with long-term studies. Hence, efforts must be made to minimize these losses. Whenever patients do not appear at the appointed time, investigations should be made immediately to allow a second date to be arranged; this date must, however, never violate the time limit fixed in advance in the study protocol. Patients whose therapy is terminated due to side-effects should be kept under observation, as the information thus obtained may furnish important points for the final interpretation of a therapeutic study. Naturally, patient drop-out cannot be entirely avoided. The inaccessible "hard core" consists of patients who refuse to continue to participate or fail to respond to calls. This type of patient drop-out should be minimized in each and every study.

Physicians' compliance

A problem related to internal quality control (and often underrated) is the compliance of physicians and their patients. Difficulties in this regard are often experienced where practising doctors and out-patients are involved in long-term studies. Meaningful cooperation with such doctors can be achieved only if they are asked to participate in the planning of the study. One should make sure that the family doctors of the patients know the obligatory therapeutic procedure and the study documents they must fill in.

Patient compliance

This depends, on the one hand, on the severity of the symptoms. For example, the compliance of pa-

tients with angina pectoris or myocardial infarction approaches 90 %; such patients suffer if they
do not take their medication. As against this,
studies have shown hypertensive patients to evidence a compliance rate of only 40 %; hypertensive
patients are often free of discomfort and may therefore forget to take their drugs regularly or feel
that they are no longer needed. Patient compliance
in such cases may be checked by questioning or by
urin-analysis (using a fluorescing agent). On the
other hand, patient compliance depends on patients'
insight into the purpose of the treatment plan and
is markedly influenced by the doctor's personality
and the doctor-patient relationship. It depends on
this relationship whether the patient is motivated
to a greater or lesser degree to stop smoking,
maintain his weight, follow a treatment schedule,
etc.. In the same study on the efficacy of exer-
cise therapy for patients suffering from myocardial infarction and angina pectoris, the controls
who received only drugs did not understand why
they were told to appear in the clinic every day
to receive their medication, as they experienced
no other medical attention (Stauch 1978).

Control of doctors' and patients' compliance is a
challenge to the imagination of the clinicians
participating in the study. It is crucial to take
the compliance factor into account, as the practical feasibility of a treatment proved to be superior depends on this.

Observational errors

The importance of comprehensive data quality control is borne out by experiments on the reliability
and reproducibility of diagnostic procedures. During the Framingham Eye Study, observational errors
were analyzed by allocating patients to examining
physicians at random and comparing diagnoses and
other findings. KAHN et al. (1975) report that
these doctors evidenced marked differences in the
frequency and severity of their diagnoses. Obvious-
ly, identical diagnostic standards would have re-

sulted in similar frequencies of diagnostic findings for all observers concerned. These observational errors occurred although a carefully prepared
study protocol existed and all participating doctors
had been trained in the required diagnostic procedures. The above authors stress that such experience
is not infrequent. In other examples, the reproducibility of diagnostic measurements was no better.
They recommend even more rigorous control of observational errors: observer training should be enhanced, the protocol enriched with respect to detail and the diagnostic procedures involved standardized as far as possible.

If a substantial amount of observational error is
found in therapeutic studies, the cogency of the
results obtained is in jeopardy. If it is known
that a number of studies on similar problems lead
to differing results, there is reason to believe
that in most of these studies no effort was made
to check up on observational errors.

3.3. Patient Recruitment and Drop-out

Ways and means
of improving
patient
recruitment

As a rule, not only in-patients take part in a
therapeutic study. A large proportion of the subjects are out-patients who are only occasionally
hospitalized or called up for specified examinations.
Hence, in recruiting patients for a study, the participating clinics depend on co-operation with practising doctors, including patient referrals. This
method of patient recruitment often leads to considerable delay in admitting the planned number of
patients to the study. Such problems may prevent
some studies from being begun and lead to premature
termination (i.e., failure) of others.

The above-mentioned patient recruitment problems
also existed in the "Coronary Primary Prevention
Trial", a multicentre study by the National Heart,
Lung and Blood Institute. An analysis of recruit-

ment via practising physicians revealed that the
weekly rate of patient admissions to the study did
not reach its pre-planned level until 40 weeks
after inception of the study. Therefore, new ways
of patient recruitment were considered (Agras,
Marshall 1979).

Exchange of information and motivation

First, weekly exchange of information between the
participating clinics was arranged for; the subject matter of these discussions consisted of the
inclusion criteria and the number of patients examined to find one patient satisfying these criteria. The discussions provided motivation and often
led to increases in the number of eligible patients.

New methods of patient recruitment

Further action taken concerned new sources for patient recruitment, viz.,
- list from blood banks
- contacts with industrial and service companies
- circulars explaining the purpose of the study,
  in which eligible persons were asked to participate
- contacts with patients who participated in previous studies
- press releases on the current study.
These measures enabled the period needed for recruiting the pre-planned number of study patients
to be markedly shortened, and were executed and
monitored by specialized staff members.

Factors having an impact on recruitment

If the recruitment practices of clinics participating in a multicentre study are to be changed, the
factors having an impact on the recruitment must
be known. For this reason, recruitment practices
of participating clinics were analyzed in a concomitant study of the "National Cooperative Gallstone Study" (Croke 1975). The recruitment activities were assessed in relation to the following
factors :
- attributes of clinics : professional reputation
  of the senior physicians (experience in therapeutic studies, research on gallstones, status

in professional societies), institutional and
administrative support of the study (providing
equipment and services), other research activities, especially basic research, type of clinic
(university, municipal or private)
- density of the population and the number of ope-
rations (cholecystectomies) performed per annum
- requirements of the study protocol
- criteria for continuation of grant(s).

Institutional support of the study

Of the four attributes of the clinics, only the
institutional and administrative support had a
beneficial influence on the number of patients recruited for the study. Population density and the
size of a clinic had no such impact: there were
signs of an inverse relationship. Clinics in small
towns recruited relatively more patients per unit
of population. The number of cholecystectomies per
year performed in a given clinic did not influence
patient recruitment.

Inclusion and exclusion criteria, forms of therapy

There was a close relationship between the requirements set out in the study protocol (especially the
inclusion and exclusion criteria) on the one hand
and patient recruitment on the other. Modification
of the eligibility criteria by including additional
age groups raised the number of study patients
allocated at random and thus shortened the study
period. Moreover, the readiness of patients to cooperate was influenced by a change in the therapeutic situation : the biopsy was eschewed in the main
study; the patients received a high or a low dose
of an anti-gallstone drug, or a placebo.

Funding as a function of numbers of patients

It was crucial for recruitment activities that both
further funding and participation in the study de-
pended on sufficient numbers of patients; after
this condition was stipulated, all clinics involved
intensified their recruitment effort, which resulted in more patients being admitted to the study.

The results of this concomitant investigation re-

futed the original belief that recruitment depends
primarily on population density and the size of a
clinic, the professional reputation of the clinicians and the research background of such clinics.

Patient drop-out due to side-effects, non-attendance and refusal	The salient causes of patient drop-out are : - side-effects requiring termination of treatment, - non-response of patients to call-ups, and - refusal to continue to take part in a study. Moreover, the drop-out rate depends on the length of the study period. Long-term studies have more drop-out than shorter ones. Drop-out from patient refusal may arise due to side-effects which may not necessitate termination from a medical point of view, but cause major patient discomfort; the latter experience was made, for example, with adjuvant therapy of breast cancer which enhanced therapeutic efficacy by the use of markedly toxic agents but caused many patients to refuse further treatment because of massive loss of hair and other symptoms (Schreml 1978).
Estimation of the drop-out rate	In estimating the drop-out rate, specific experience is required. Side-effects of therapies are usually known. A study should never be begun if a considerable incidence of severe side-effects must be expected. During one controlled study on rheumatoid arthritis, treatment of 50% of the patients of the study group had to be terminated because of severe side-effects. In the control group, only 15 of 53 patients tolerated the full duration of the experiment, as the condition of placebo-treated patients worsened so markedly that an effective drug had to be introduced. Such studies may be also ethically indefensible (Dreher 1978). The amount of drop-out from non-response or refusal depends on patient control. Drop-out is often due to negligence, such as insufficient motivation of the patients to cooperate until the end of the study is reached, or carelessness in keeping the address file. In addition to this, there are uncontrollable factors contributed by the patients. Especially

when long-term studies are planned, special care
must be taken to organize a meaningful follow-up.

The expected drop-out rate due to known factors
must be taken into account in determining the number of patients to be recruited. However, there may
be limitations in this regard due to constraints
on patient availability, e.g., in studies on rare
diseases.

3.4. Termination of Therapeutic Studies

A controlled clinical study conforms to accepted ethical standards only
if currently existing experience supports the hypothesis of equivalence
of the therapies being compared. It may become necessary to stop a study
if preliminary results are found to the effect that one of these therapies is superior; the same action must be required following undesirable
side-effects, major patient drop-out or publication of findings of other
researchers. With multicentre studies, specific precautions for such
cases must be taken into consideration at the very outset, i.e., during
the planning phase. Moreover, not only premature but also regular termination requires a number of decisions and measures concerning the patients
and doctors involved in a study. Moreover, data analysis and evaluation
and publication of results should be pre-planned in time.

Decision-
making on
premature
termination

The decision on premature termination of a multicentre study is made by the chief investigator in
cooperation with the principle investigators in
the clinics. For this purpose, the results of current evaluations must be presented to the coordinating centre from time to time. We recommend asking
an independent advisory body to participate in the
deliberations preceding a decision. More detail on
eventual premature termination should be set out
in the study protocol and/or the experimental design.

Interim
results
and the course
of a study

If the design of a study stipulates sequential analysis or monitoring at regular intervals, this implies a necessity of deciding on continuation or
termination of a study at fixed points in time. We

know from experience with controlled clinical
studies that the presentation of interim results
often fails to furnish a base for clear-cut decision on continuation or termination of a study.
MEIER pointed out that evidence of superiority of
a form of therapy from statistical significance
tests alone is not enough. He is in favour of a
flexible stopping rule with a "maximum acceptable"
and a "least interesting" difference. This method
calls for termination after a fixed period, if
either one of the therapeutic alternatives has
reached the "maximum acceptable" or neither therapy reaches the "least interesting" difference.
The study is to be continued as long as this minimum is attained by one of the therapeutic methods
(Meier 1979).

**Results of
other research;
prejudice and
interest; the
advisory body
and its
members**

The attempt to define criteria for termination
allowing as rational decisions as are possible is
overshadowed by the problem of the advisory body
being influenced in decision-finding by other factors. These include - especially - results of domestic or foreign research done by others becoming
known in the meantime, which are either in favour
or opposed to the therapies under study. Such results may be clear-cut or more or less equivocal.
In the latter case, it depends also in interests
and prejudices among the members of the advisory
body - and on who these members are - which decision is finally reached in an individual case. "Independent" advisory bodies are hence no guarantee
that controlled clinical studies are terminated at
the proper time. This is especially serious in the
case of multicentre studies terminated without conclusive results, due to the amount of planning and
organizational effort lost and the unrecoverable
expense.

**Action to
be taken upon
termination
of studies**

KLIMT and CANNER have analyzed a number of multi-
centre studies: "University Group Diabetes Program",
"Coronary Drug Project Aspirin Study", "Aspirin
Myocardial Infarction Study", and "Diabetic Retino-

pathy Study". The recommendations set out in the following are derived from the above-mentioned authors (Klimt, Canner 1979).

Termination of individual patients

If treatment of individual patients is terminated on account of health risks, a study is not endangered as long as the criteria for such termination are unequivocal and reproducible; important experience in this regard should be published. During the further course of the study, one should make use of opportunities to review such decisions on termination.

Premature termination of a therapeutical study

If the entire study is prematurely terminated, all persons involved should be informed, and the patients should be observed in the time following the event with a view to monitoring possible effects of such termination. If only one of several therapy groups of a study is terminated, it is desirable that the patients belonging to this group are examined as stipulated in the study protocol until the study is regularly ended. The patients should not be transferred to another group. If because of unexpected events an important change in the study protocol has to be made the ongoing of the study depends on developing, in cooperation with all involved, a strategy leading to a new consensus as to how to proceed in the future. This includes informing the patients on the results thus far, consent of suitable patients to the new therapy plan, having the coordinating centre give the doctors conducting the treatment the information they need, informing the public and disucssion of results in the scientific community.

End of studies

The possible outcomes of a study are :
- a clinically positive effect of the therapy under study
- no clear-cut decision as to its effects, i.e, the results do not show sufficient superiority of the therapy to the ones it was compared with.

At the end of a study, the further treatment of the patients according to the results obtained must be ensured, preferably by recommendations to the physicians entrusted with the care for these patients. In addition to this, the data on the patients must be updated. Information on adherence to experimental design (e.g., double-blind tests and regular medical care) should be raised. Further measures concern monitoring of after-effects on patients who dropped out of the study and reviewing the feasibility of long-term follow-up of study patients as to mortality, especially if there is any suspicion of carcinogenesis.

Preparation and evaluation of the data

The coordinating centre should continue to exist after the end of the study proper. Data preparation and evaluation requires the fixing of a cut-off date, after which no more data are admitted for documentation and evaluation. At the end of the study, it must be ensured that suitable persons are appointed for the task of preparing and publishing the results; only such appointees should be considered that have participated in planning and implementing the study. A writing committee should be charged with preparing the text of the publications. Last but not least, it must be settled where the study documents are stored and what should happen to drugs and apparatus no longer needed. Regarding the storage of patient-related documents, the provisions on data protection must be adhered to.

Publication of the results of a study

These results should first be made known to all participants in the study. It is not advisable to publish such results in the press before a scientific publication of these results has appeared. Press releases and presentation of results at scientific meetings should, wherever possible, follow and not precede publication in a scientific journal.

4. Assessment of Therapeutic Methods

In the methodology of therapeutic studies, the effectiveness criteria
for therapeutic methods are considered to be well-established. As a
rule, the literature contains only the point that such criteria must
be exactly defined and amenable to operationalization, i.e., measurable. However, the choice of the "proper" or suitable effectiveness
criteria is often extremely problematical, especially if diseases that
do not endanger life stand for the fore.

A further problem is the question of the interrelationship of a therapy
and the outcome measured. The effectiveness of a treatment is not independent of the way it was performed and the context in which it took
place.

4.1. Selection and Measurement of Effectiveness Criteria

Mortality
and
morbidity

For the assessment of therapeutic success, effectiveness criteria such as death, survival time and
the incidence of medical complications (subsequent
illnesses and severe side-effects) stand right-
fully to the fore. However, the assessment of the
quality of life requires subjective and less
"hardened" variables as additional criteria. This
is especially true of illnesses that, in general,
do not endanger life, e.g., rheumatic and mental
diseases. For the patients, subjective discomfort,
overall condition and social integration are frequently more important than physiological parameters. A realistic assessment of therapeutic
success must take life-quality aspects into
account over and above the mortality and morbidity criteria. Thus, for assessment of different
types of breast cancer surgery, the psychological
and social impact on the patients should be duly
considered.

The spectrum
of effectivenes
criteria

Comprehensive assessment of therapies requires observation with respect to effectiveness criteria
at different levels. BROOK et al. (1979) have

analyzed the literature and the current studies
with respect to such criteria. The following criteria were listed as related to four levels:
physiological status, physical functioning, mental
and social health (Ware et al. 1980).

o Physiological status (Brook et al. 1977, p.83)

"- functioning of organ systems : level of function, abnormality in function, external
   support of function

 - morbidity : primary (study condition), comor-
   bidity (level of symptoms, progression of
   disease, prognosis)

 - mortality/longevity : life expectancy, death."

o Physical functioning (Stewart et al. 1978, p.1)

"- self-care activities : feeding, bathing,
   dressing, and going to the toilet

 - mobility: getting around indoors, outdoors,
   or in the community

 - physical activities: running, walking, using
   stairs, lifting and moving one's body in a
   variety of ways

 - role activities: activities typical for an
   individual of a specified age and social role
   (work, school or housework)

 - household activities: housekeeping duties
   (major role activity for some and minor role
   activity for others)

 - leisure activities: hobbies, clubs, church,
   sports etc."

o Mental health (Ware et al. 1979, pp.1 - 5)

 - depression

 - absence of positive well-being

 - anxiety

 - loss of control over feelings, thought and
   behavior

o Social health (Donald et al. 1978, pp.3 - 4)

"- work (supervisors, coworkers, subordinates,
   work-achievements, work tasks)

 - family (spouse support, children, kinship
   support)

 - social life (friendships, leisure, community
   activities, opportunities to play, hobbies)

- financial adequacy
- social rituals (religious life, parties)
- personal community life (warmth, trust, confidants)
- privacy (personal time, quiet time)
- value-identity support (living preferred life-style, personal philosophy, sense of achievement, recognition, new experiences)
- sexual satisfaction".

The above catalogue shows the spectrum of conceivable criteria in general terms, which must be reified in accordance with the problem to be solved by a given therapeutic study. At the physiological level, this reification is given by the disease under observation, the treatments assessed and the existing diagnostic and prognostic experience on the subject. Establishing relevant problem-oriented criteria is more difficult at the other levels, as considering physical, mental and social impairments is relatively new in medicine. Hence, experience and knowledge as to disease-specific criteria is lacking.

This problem can be solved by submitting the above list to the doctors and asking them to select the criteria needed for a comprehensive assessment of the outcome of the treatment for given conditions. One example is reported by BROOK et al. (1977) for breast cancer surgery: the doctors all agreed that an assessment of therapeutic success should be supported not only by physiological criteria but also - and more so - by data on disturbed sex relations, depressive conditions and attitutes toward the body.

Effectiveness criteria must be as specific as possible at all levels, as this is necessary to provide unequivocal disease-treatment relationship constructs. Hence, one should, when choosing effectiveness criteria for therapeutic studies prefer

such physical, psychological and social criteria
as are well founded in experienced fact. In addition to this, the length of the observation period
has an impact on the selection of suitable effectiveness criteria. The probability of occurrence of
given criteria is assessed differently in long-
term investigations than in shorter studies.

Weighing of
effectiveness
criteria

Whenever the degree of therapeutic success is
assessed comprehensively by using criteria at
different levels, the problems of interdependence
and of weighing the individual criteria arise: it
must be made clear in which way the criteria are
interrelated, and whether they are all equally important as to therapeutic success. The relationship
between criteria from different levels may be very
complex. The ideal case in which all criteria vary
uniformly during the course of treatment is not
the rule in clinical practice. An improvement
according to one criterion may co-exist with an
unchanged condition according to another. Such situations may be expected to occur the most frequently whenever there is little or no correlation between the above-mentioned levels. For example, psy-
chopharmacological and psychotherapeutic studies
meet with such problems (Benkert 1978; von Cranach
1978). The effects of psychotropic drugs at the
biochemical level are not unequivocally related
with corresponding changes at the psychopathologi-
cal level. Psychotherapy may be effective on the
latter level without changing the social behaviour
of patients in the desired manner.

As a rule, the different levels and the criteria
selected at each of these have differing degrees
of importance in the assessment of therapeutic
effectiveness. Mortality criteria come to the fore
where life-endangering diseases are concerned. However, physiological criteria must not always be
more important than physical, psychological and
social impairments. This holds true not only for

mental and emotional diseases but also for organic
diseases. A good example for the latter are rheumatic illnesses, in which subjective symptoms are
more important indicators for therapy assessment
than objective findings such as X-ray photographs
(Ströbel 1978). Doctors understandably tend to put
more significance on physiological criteria than
on other impairments. This may be justified in many
cases, but may result in neglecting the patients'
point of view. When comprehensive, multilevel therapy assessment is called for, it should be warran-
ted that it is truly comprehensive not only from
the physicians' but also from the patients' point
of view. Hence, the standpoint of the patients must
be duly considered whenever one attempts to weigh
the criteria.

Measurement of
effectiveness
criteria

Effectiveness criteria are suited to therapeutic
studies only if such criteria are amenable to
operationalization or measurement. We require unequivocal methods enabling the criteria to be
measured. However, if the criteria are non-physio-
logical, cooperation and/or verbal information by
and/or from the patients is indispensable. The
differentiation between "hard" and "soft" data in
medicine is due to this fact.

The best way of raising "soft" criteria is asking
the patients by means of questionnaires; for reasons
of economy, a self-administered questionnaire should
be used with which patients can work independently.
The questionnaires used for such data acquisition
need not, as a rule, be developed from scratch: one
should, wherever possible, use existing questionnaires. A profusion of such questionnaires which
are, in general, either based on index- or on scale-
constructions (Blalock 1974) may be found in the
bibliography of the Clearinghouse on Health Indexes
(NCHS) and in STEWART et al. (1978), WARE et al.
(1979) and DONALD et al. (1978). For the assessment
of the psychological level we refer especially to

the collection of measurements published by CIPS
(1981) and by GUY (1976).

4.2. Additional Influencing Factors

Quality of
Medical
Care

The efficacy of a therapy also depends on the
quality of the treatment and on the situation in
which such treatment is applied. This implies that
statements on therapeutic effectiveness are not
absolute, but conditional propositions. In each
case, the conditions and/or standards of patient
care must be set out in addition to the effectiveness found (Brook et al. 1977). Controlled clinical
therapeutic studies test such effectiveness in an
experimental situation. For medical practice, however, effectiveness in real, not experimental,
situations is the point. This may result in the
following: a given therapy is shown to be effective
in a controlled clinical trial but fails to be
so in practice, as the practical situation allows
only sub-optimal conditions for this therapy (as
opposed to optimal ones during the study). This
problem may occur if applying the therapy requires
very specialized personnel and/or intensive care
for the patients. If it is the aim of therapeutic
studies to give recommendations for the mass application of therapies, the trial situation must have
a context approaching the reality of medical practice. Otherwise, it should be recommended that the
therapy should not be widely applied, but rather
be restricted to certain centres.

Therapist,
patient and
environmental
variables

A scientific causal model is presupposed in controlled clinical therapeutic studies. This implies
a causal relationship between the therapy and the
course of a given illness. However, if complex
interactions obtain between the therapy and therapist, patient and environment variables as in mental disorders, and if the impact of therapy on the
course of the illness cannot be separated in a

clear-cut manner from the above-mentioned inter-
vening variables, the implementation of controlled
clinical therapeutic studies becomes difficult,
and/or the results of such trials present problems
in interpretation. In evaluation research, methods
derived from models in social science exist which
lead us to recommend for such cases that studies
be performed on the overall situation surrounding
the therapy in order to find out, first of all,
which effects are therapy-specific and which are
not. Such studies must be based on a comparison
(or comparisons), and will profit from applying
standard principles of controlled therapeutic
studies (Guttentag, Struening 1975).

5. General Boundary Conditions of Therapeutic Studies

The controlled clinical study as such has raised a controversy on ethics which has now lasted for some years. This chapter deals with the arguments for and against such trials and with the relevant provisions of law as applicable to therapeutic studies.

Moreover, the following contains an appraisal of possible incentives for increasing scientists' interest in therapeutic studies. For a physician aspiring after an academic reputation, work on problems regarding the scientific basis of therapies promises more rewards than may be expected from applying himself to questions involving the testing of therapeutic principles which already exist. The relative worth and the success of this type of research depends on the extent to which its attractiveness can be enhanced in the context of medical science.

5.1. Ethical and Legal Problems

Object of
controversy

Controlled clinical trials differ from other types of studies in that randomization is used, i.e., chance allocation of the patients to different treatment groups or therapeutic alternatives. Such randomization confers on such studies the status of experiments enabling causal inferences to be made. According to current thinking, the superiority of a therapy is felt to be really established only if shown by a randomized clinical study. Such randomization is ethically and legally proper if the therapeutic alternatives are deemed to be equivalent. Critics argue that the decision on existence or non-existence of such equivalence if often very difficult to make, with the consequence of the ethical permissibility of randomization becoming problematical. Moreover, there are doubts whether the gain in knowledge is, in all cases concerned, greater than in non-randomized studies.

Problematical
equivalence
of therapies

It depends both on the amount and the kind of existing knowledge whether therapies are deemed to be equivalent. As a rule, some experience as to their effectiveness exists. Except for the special case of drug testing, the therapies involved are always such as have been allowed to be marketed and thus must already have fulfilled specific effectiveness criteria. It is not the aim of a controlled clinical study to prove the efficacy of a therapy as such, but to show the superiority of a given therapy to a standard therapy or to a therapy taken for comparison ("control"). Non-equivalence of therapies is, therefore, in evidence (for proponents of randomized studies) only if knowledge pre-exists that implies a reasonable expectation of the superiority of one of the therapies in question. CHALMERS (1975) who strongly advocates randomized studies, sees a solution of the problem in randomizing at the outset, i.e., from the moment on, in which the first patient receives the new therapy. CHALMERS opposes pilot studies without randomization, as these create a tendency to find reasons to expect a specific therapy to be the superior one. This plausible proposal creates, however, a new problem: if it is strictly followed, patients may enjoy the advantage of a new therapy only if they are willing to take part in randomized studies. FREIREICH and GEHAN, outstanding critics of this procedure, call it a "cruel irony" (1979, p. 293).

Legal practice

A really satisfactory solution of the problem of therapeutic equivalence does not exist up to now. Legal practice, e.g., in the Federal Republic of Germany uses the supposition that not every kind of previous information precludes a controlled clinical study. The decision depends on the weight of information on superiority and on the feasibility of applying such information (from foreign studies) to the case in question. A mere conjecture as to probable superiority does not reach the threshold of penal relevance. The most important precondition is that the patient is fully informed as to the experiment and its design. Moreover, he must, before taking part in randomized studies, know all relevant therapeutic alternatives (Deutsch 1979; Linzbach 1980; von Bar, Fischer 1980).

Limited gain in knowledge by randomized trials

FREIREICH and GEHAN (1979) doubt the gain in knowledge from randomized studies mainly by pointing out that such studies do not guarantee that unequivocal statements can be made as to the superiority of a therapy: sometimes, mutually contradictory results are found. This cannot be solely put down to avoidable methodological mistakes in the design of the studies in question. In fact, it is found again and again that the elimination of confounding variables - which is the purpose of randomization - cannot be fully achieved. The experimental character of such studies can be realized only in a limited way in field situations such as the clinical setting. FREIREICH and GEHAN maintain that the randomized clinical study as a technique is only one method among others with specific advantages and drawbacks. Other study types not requiring randomization, such as "historical controls", are available. Further, present therapeutic knowledge has originated from other sources than from randomized studies.

However, non-randomized studies differ in epistemiological value from randomized ones. If we follow FREIREICH's and GEHAN's (1979) demand and renounce the randomization technique, we will give away also the opportunity existing in principle of proving causal relationships.

Clinical research and ethical norms

The above-described controversy on the ethics of randomized studies is only one aspect of the ethically implications of therapeutic studies. The basic principles on human experiments in medicine are laid down in the Nuremberg Code and in the 1975 revision of the Declaration of Helsinki. LEVINE and LEBACQZ (1979) have derived six ethical norms for clinical research on humans from these basic

principles:
- a good research design
- a balance of harm and benefit
- competence of the investigator
- informed consent
- equitable selection of subjects
- compensation for research-related injury.

Underlying principles of beneficence, nonmaleficence, respecting persons and justice

The investigators must be competent and the aims and methods of the research must be meaningful and proper, if a human benefit is to result and harm to be avoided. These demands on research and investigators are also a necessary condition for the prevention of abuse of people taking part in clinical studies, and are helpful in providing for due adherence to the norm giving individuals a right to self-determination. The latter is specifically expressed in the norm of fully informed patient consent. As it is possible to refuse to take part in a study, this norm also follows principles of beneficience and nonmaleficience. The norm of equitable selection of subjects aims at preventing certain social groups from being subjected to more experimentation than others; this is intended to protect "dependent" groups such as children, prison inmates and committed incompetents. By compensating subjects for research related injury, it is taken into account that society is the beneficiary of research and that, therefore, society must indemnify individuals volunteering for a study for eventual injury sustained. The last two of the six norms listed above reflect the norms of justice and/or distributing goods and evils fairly.

Application of principles to patient recruitment and informed consent

LEVINE and LEBACQZ (1979) illustrate the application of the principles using the example of patient recruitment and informed consent in therapeutic studies. They find that it is incompatible with the prinicple of justice to recruit a higher proportion of VA patients than of private patients

for controlled clinical studies. This would be so
if VA patients could enjoy the advantage of a new
therapy only if they were willing to take part in
a randomized study, whereas private patients with
their better facilities of freely choosing doctors
and hospitals obtained this new therapy without
taking part in a therapeutic study.

LEVINE and LEBACQZ (1979) state further, that it
is necessary to give the patients complete information on randomization and therapeutic alternatives, especially whenever substantial interests
of such patients are involved. The legal provisions (DHEW Regulations) are not clear-cut, as no
rules on the actual extent of the information to
be given are set out. Furthermore, there is the
possibility of severe illnesses in which information and consent may be omitted to avoid endanger-
ing therapeutic success. In such cases, the principles of beneficience and nonmaleficience are
given priority over the right to individual self-
determination (principle of respecting persons)
which would require such information (and consent).
CHALMERS (1967) uses this argument in maintaining
that detailed patient information on therapeutic
alternatives is not required. He stresses that
non-jeopardization of the success of treatment must
take precedence. In cases involving equivalent
therapies, the benefit for the patient is the same,
notwithstanding which treatment is decided on.
LEVINE and LEBACQZ object to this : "equivalent"
therapies from the doctors' standpoint must not
be so for the patients. They give an impressive
example: the comparison of radical mastectomy with
wide excision in the treatment of early breast
cancer. From the doctors' standpoint, the therapies are equivalent because both procedures have
the same long-term morbidity and mortality rates.
There is no such equivalence from the women's
point of view, as far as other criteria are important for her - in this case, the fact that re-

stricted surgery was of a less "mutilating character". As substantial interests of the patients are
involved, consent to participation in a randomized
study should be asked for only after full and detailed information on the alternatives of surgical
procedure; moreover, patients refusing to take
part in the study should be given the opportunity
to receive the operation they want.

**Problems
concerning
patient
consent**

Even if a patient is fully informed, his consent
to taking part in a randomized study may be ethically problematical: in some cases it can be as-
sumed that a patient is not in a situation allowing free decision. The illness situation fosters
dependence, anxiety and susceptibility to sugges-
tion; this in turn influences the doctor-patient
relationship and the communication between the two
parties. If we further consider that patients are,
as a rule, medical laymen and therefore cannot
enter into a conversation on equal terms with
their doctors, we must doubt the ability of the
patients to make free decisions. FLETCHER (1979)
has studied these problems in detail and recommends
that consent to taking part in a randomized study
should be elicited not by the doctor conducting
the treatment alone, but through a "consent committee" acting as an independent third party me-
diating between the doctor and his patient and making sure that the patient is capable of a free decision.

**Permissibility
of physicians'
therapeutic
action**

The pertinent legal provisions of the West German
penal code and of the West German civil code, on
causing bodily harm are also applicable to therapeutic studies, with and without the use of drugs
(Deutsch 1979; Linzbach, 1980; Bar, Fischer 1980).
Paramedical measures and psychotherapy are included under these laws, which stipulate the consent
of the patient or his legal representative after
due information. The doctor may practically go as
far as the patient's consent allows him to. The

right of the patient to self-determination does
not include a right to unjustified consent, i.e.,
consent to unreasonable risks such as an unnecessary risk of death. Legally, risking death is allowed only if therapeutic strategies are applicable
to life-endangering illnesses in such a way that
an unfavourable outcome threatens the patient's
life. The informed consent of the patient may be
eschewed in cases of severe illness if the success
of treatment is thereby jeopardized and no counter-
manding will of this patient is seen to exist. The
administration of justice presupposes competent
patients and their expected decision after due information for such situations.

The drug law on clinical tests

The provisions of the German drug law on clinical
tests (Hasskarl, Kleinsorge 1979) are relevant to
therapeutic studies if a non-licensed drug is to
be tested, or a licensed one tested in situations
not covered by such license (such as new indications). The law stipulates that the test risk must
be reasonable (as seen from experiments on animals)
and that furthermore a concrete therapeutic benefit must be expected for the patients taking part
in the study. Clinical trials on ill persons require oral consent before witnesses, and such trials
on healthy subjects need written consent. Subjects
and patients must be personally free: this excludes
inmates of prisons and mental hospitals. The study
must be made under the supervision of an experienced physician. The law draws special attention to
the requirement that sufficient pharmacological
and toxicological testing must be completed before
a new drug is administered to humans. Because of
possible side-effects, a special insurance policy
must be taken out. In this regard, it is disputed
whether, in addition to the above, also pharmacological and toxicological documentation must be
deposited (Lewandowski 1979).

The law

According to the West German Law on Data Protec-

on data
protection

tion (Deutsch 1979) the answer to the question
whether data may be stored and transmitted for use
in research depends on patient consent. Any oral
expression of consent is to be regarded as specific.
Any multicentre study involving non-anonymous patient data depends on the following acts of consent:
- consent to the study
- consent to having data raised under professional
  secrecy passed on to third parties
- consent to data storage and transmission.
In practice, such consent may be given by the patient, to whom the project must be previously explained, by a simple declaration or an equivalent
act (such as a nod).

Special
provisions
and problems
concerning
the mentally
ill

In psychiatry, the existence of patients incapable
of consent or reasening gives rise to unusual legal
problems. The current practice of substituting personal decisions by those of a legally appointed
representative, of appointing guardians and óf
court-ordered committal of patients to mental hospitals is unsatisfactory, and leads, in many cases,
to discrimination against the mentally ill as compared with physically ill patients. For participation of psychiatric patients in therapeutic studies,
it is, above all, necessary to regulate the guardianship and committal procedures in such a manner
as to ensure that the consent required is given in
a formally and materially satisfactory way. The unfavourable consequences of guardianship could be
avoided by ensuring that only duly qualified persons are appointed guardians: this would free the
doctors treating such patients from the double responsibility for both their own and the patient's
interests (Helmchen, Müller-Oerlinghausen 1978).

Whenever testing new drugs is the object of therapeutic studies, the West German drug law specifically prohibits the inclusion of committee patients
in such studies.

Placebos, randomization, blind and double-blind procedure	The West German drug law does not regulate the administering of placebos. The provisions of this law relate only to the drugs tested. For placebo experiments, the law on physicians' therapeutic action is the proper criterion: a placebo experiment is permissible if therapeutically meaningful. For randomized studies and blind and double-blind procedures, the most important requirement is the informed consent of the patients to the experiment(s) as planned. Patients should know about all the therapeutic alternatives involved (Deutsch 1979).

5.2. Incentives for Participation in Therapeutic Studies

Competition with "basis research" and lack of sponsorship	Therapeutic studies are a relatively new field of research in the history of medical science. A review of the past decade shows increasing importance of this new speciality on the one hand and hesitation on the part of young scientists to commit themselves to this field on the other. This may be explained in part by the traditional scale of values in medical science. According to which basic research - including basic clinical research - is a better opportunity for acquiring academic prestige than work on problems concerning the quality and efficacy of medical care. A second reason for such preferences is the situation regarding research sponsorship. The Federal Government's Program on Promoting Research and Development in the Service of Health (BMFT 1978) is the first official party in West Germany to take responsibility for free promotion of research in the field of therapeutic studies. Up to then, such studies were funded almost exclusively by the drug industry which implemented the studies in cooperation with clinics. Understandably, drug testing and other pharmacological studies stood to the fore in this connection.
Little opportunity	A third reason for the above-mentioned reluctance may be found in the field under discussion. The

for personal image-building	implementation of therapeutic studies, especially multicentre projects, gives little opportunity for personal image-building. COCHRANE has put this very aptly: "A randomized clinical trial is great fun for the coordinator but can be very boring for the scattered physicians filling in the forms" (Cochrane 1973, p.24). It takes, as a rule, years until first results are published, and such publications appear not under a single name, but under several ones or the title of the research project.
Authorship, independent publications, spin-off research	RELMAN proposes that only such persons be named as authors or co-authors who have made considerable contributions to the planning and implementation of a study, whereas other co-workers should be mentioned in footnotes in an appendix (Relman 1979). In addition to this, MEINERT and HAWKINS (1979) feel it to be commendable to limit the number of joint publications to specific cases and to give individuals the opportunity of writing publications on special subjects. With large-scale cooperative studies, it is often feasible to link smaller research projects on interesting marginal problems or specialized questions to such a study. The smaller projects would need only little additional personnel or expense and could be handled in the course of the general implementation of the study proper. According to RELMAN, such "spin-off research", which could enhance the willingness of young scientists to participate in studies, is feasible in flexibly organized research, and should be taken into consideration by research sponsors.
Funding the planning of studies	Studies, and especially multicentre ones, require comprehensive and detailed planning, which in turn needs time and money. The willingness to participate in such studies is often lacking because no funds are available for the preparation of plans and protocols for these projects. Institutions sponsoring research should not maintain that planning a study and preparing the requisite protocol

are preconditions to be fulfilled by project applicants, as the work entailed in these activities
is, as a rule, on an unusually large scale; one
example is extensive travel for meetings needed
whenever hospitals at different locations participate in a study.

**Flexibility
in funding**

A further problem in sponsorship of therapeutic
studies is posed by the funding envisioned. It is
often the rule that funds for participating clinics are a function of the number of patients subjected to the study procedure. This leads to in-
creased recruitment activity but also entails a
risk that the inclusion criteria are not always
followed with sufficient care. Unfavourable consequences could possibly be prevented by "mixed"
funding: fixed funds are budgeted for the personnel involved in the study, without reference
to the number of patients taking part in the study.
The manpower needed for studies is usually under-
estimated, as is the time required. The funding
should be so flexible in time that "bungling" of
data acquisition near the end of the study is not
encouraged.

**Avoidance of
"red tape"**

Wherever multicentre studies are made, central
facilities are needed for the central managing
committee, for data analysis, quality control,
laboratory tests, etc., which must, in turn, be
managed. If a study is randomized, a number of
committees exist due to the ethical and legal implications of the project (ethics committee, consent committee, etc.); this results in even more
administrative work. This has the possible effect
of creating a bureaucratic structure immobilizing
innovative research. This raises the question of
the optimum organizational structure of cooperative studies and the optimal size of such studies.
However, one should also ponder whether the study
type chosen and the expense it entails is in a
reasonable relation to the problem to be solved.

5.3. Measures to Improve and Promote Development of The Speciality of Therapeutic Studies

Continued development of the methodology of therapeutic studies

Specific incentives for participation in therapeutic studies and full funding of the same are not a sufficient foundation for medical evaluation research as a field in its own right. There is a need for a number of specific measures calculated to enhance professionalism and to develop this field of research. First of all, REINERT and HAWKINS (1979) call for advancement of the methodology of therapeutic studies by means of specialized research sponsorship. The existing methods are primarily keyed to problems in pharmacology and to testing individual modes of therapy. Methodological difficulties are encountered in the validation of complex therapeutic strategies involving combinations and sequences of surgery, radiotherapy, chemotherapy, physical, social and psychotherapy. Methodological advancement should, hence, be primarily concerned with the analysis of multivariate problems.

Structural improvements in communications

Other measures concern the exchange of scientific information by qualified publications on therapeutic studies, systematic documentation of all current and completed research projects, and above all by direct reporting on experience within professional societies, at special meetings and other events.

Missing items in publications on therapeutic studies

Analyses of the literature have shown that the quality of recent publications on therapeutic studies and their methodology is not quite what one could wish. MOSTELLER (1979) has analyzed 107 publications on therapeutic studies in the fields of surgery and anaesthesiology and mentions the following instances of inadequate reporting. Frequently, one or more of the following items are left undescribed:
- the concrete procedural details on randomization
- the way patient consent was obtained, and the problems (if any) encountered in this connection
- the details of the techniques used in statistical analysis

- the entire body of data obtained (no descriptive statistics)
- the power of the statistical tests performed (i.e., the degree of conclusiveness)
- selection bias, if any, in the results as presented: it is not made clear whether the entire result of the study or only a selected, especially interesting partial result is set out.

Defects of the methodological literature

SCHOOLMAN (1979) has analyzed literature samples on the methodology of therapeutic studies taken from the MEDLINE (National Library of Medicine) documentation system. He finds that
- in general, more literature on the subject is needed
- standardization of terms and their synonyms would be worthwhile
- catchwords for literature research on methods require improvement.

SCHOOLMAN recommends, in addition to the above, that a documentation on study protocols should be established.

"Journal of Therapeutic Studies" needed

During the National Conference on Clinical Trials Methodology held in Bethesda,MD, on October 3 - 4, 1977 (ROTH, GORDON 1979) the above-mentioned problems with publications on therapeutic studies were attributed to the fact that a specialized journal dealing with the subject does not, as yet, exist. It was maintained, that the requisite comprehensive and detailed reports on therapeutic studies - complete with comment on problems and boundary conditions - would find no room in large-circulation medical journals. In these, special issues dealing with the subject would be conceivable; however, an independent organ for such publications would be more meaningful. The latter solution would, in all probability, not be feasible in the Federal Republic of Germany, as the number of subscribers would remain too small, even considering the potential of other German-speaking

countries. A first step in the proper direction
would be concentrating publications on certain
medical journals. Extensive reports could be published independently as monographs.

Criteria for
publications
on therapeutic
studies

In order to avoid the above-mentioned inadequacies
of publications on therapeutic studies, MEINERT
(1978, p. J-118) recommends a catalogue of criteria for authors, editors and scientific publishers.
Publications on this subject should deal with the
following points:
"- the source of funding for the study and an indication of whether results reported represent
   a subgroup of a larger unreported set of data
 - a listing of the treatment groups studied and
   the rationale for the choice
 - a description of the method of treatment allocation, including a description of the level
   of masking for treatment allocations (i.e.,
   issued unmasked, single or double masked)
 - the safeguards used in the study to protect
   patient rights to informed consent and privacy
 - patient exclusion criteria
 - patient admission criteria
 - rationale for the number of patients studied,
   including statement of the assumptions used in
   the sample size calculation if one was made
 - statement of the length of time required to
   complete enrolment in the study
 - a description of the population(s) from which
   patients were selected
 - a description of the baseline and follow-up
   examination schedule
 - a definition of the key endpoint or response
   variable of the study
 - descriptive information on the baseline comparability of the treatment groups
 - the number of patients assigned to each treatment group
 - the level of compliance achieved in each treatment group
 - the number of patients followed to the end of

the study or to death
- the number of deceased patients
- the number of patients unable or unwilling to
  return for follow-up examinations including a
  count of the number who have been lost to follow-
  up and could not be located at the end of the
  study
- a description of the methods of analysis used
  in the report
- a description of tests of significance used, including an indication of whether or not p values
  reported resulted from a single or multiple evaluations of the data
- a discussion of the power of the observed sample
  size to detect a treatment difference of the
  size observed if the difference is regarded as
  insignificant."

**Development of
a methodology
of errors**

Some points might well be added to the above list
of criteria and some may possibly be done without.
It is by no means the purpose of the list to make
inflexible rules for publications; the meaning of
this catalogue of criteria is to acquaint prospective authors with such criteria so that they may
endeavour to set out the type of their study, its
course in time, the problems encountered, including undesirable experiences, as plainly and completely as needed. Such publications should help
avoid unnecessary mistakes, so that neophytes in
the field of therapeutic studies need not always
experience the pitfalls of such research by themselves (Lasagna 1979). In the further development
of the methodology of therapeutic studies, it is
important to include the methology of errors based
on recent studies and concrete experience.

**Possibility
of direct
exchange of
experience**

Direct exchange of experience is especially important for the professionalization of a research
field. As a rule, therapeutic studies require an
interdisciplinary mode of work. This means that,
along with the physicians from different medical
specialities, methodologists, epidemiologists,

psychologists, social scientists - and, when occasion arises, also lawyers - are all given a special part in the planning, implementation and evaluation of the studies; the direct exchange of experience referred to above must be organized in such a way as to take this interdisciplinary structure into account. It is an open question whether such exchange is best implemented through a special scientific society or through other channels. One alternative would be to institutionalize the exchange of information in connection with specified research promotion programmes. For West Germany, the Federal Government programme on Promoting Research and Development in the Service of Health (BMFT 1978) could provide such facilities.

The organization of professional education, both basic and advanced, should be duly considered. This holds true both for those who are primarily interested in the new field of therapeutic studies and for other participators in such studies whose central research interest is elsewhere.

References

Chapter 1

Althauser, R.P., D.B. Rubin: The computerized construction of a matched sample. American Journal of Sociology 76 (1970) 325 - 346

Armitage, P.: Restricted sequential procedures. Biometrica 44 (1957) 9 - 26

Armitage, P.: Statistical methods in medical research. Oxford: Blackwell 1971

Armitage, P.: Sequential medical trials, 2nd edition. Oxford: Blackwell 1975

Atkins, H.: Controlled trials. British Medical Journal 1 (1966) 1101 - 1109

Boston Collaborative Drug Surveillance Program: Regular aspirin intake and acute myocardial infarction. British Medical Journal 1 (1974) 440 - 443

Breslow, N.E.: Regression analysis of the odds ratio: A method for retrospective studies. Biometrics 32 (1976) 409 - 416

Breslow, N.E., N.E. Day, K.T. Halvorsen, R.L. Prentice, C. Sabai: Estimation of multiple relative risk functions in machted case-control-studies. American Journal of Epidemiology 108 (1978) 299 - 307

Bross, I.: Sequential medical plans. Biometrics 8 (1952) 188 - 205

Bross, I.: Misclassification in 2 x 2 tables. Biometrics 9 (1954) 478 - 486

Bross, I.: How case-for-case matching can improve design efficiency. American Journal of Epidemiology 89 (1969) 359 - 363

Cochran, W.G.: Matching in analytical studies. American Journal of Public Health 43 (1953) 684 - 691

Cochran, W.G.: The planning of observational studies in human populations. Journal of the Royal Statistical Society, Series A 128 (1965) 234 - 266

Cochran, W.G.: Sampling techniques, 2nd edition. New York, London: Wiley 1963

Cochran, W.G., G.M. Cox: Experimental designs, 2nd edition. New York, London, Sidney: Wiley 1957

Cornfield, J.: A statistical problem arising from retrospective studies. Proceedings of the Third Berkeley Symposium 4 (1956) 135 - 148

Cornfield, J.: Recent methodological contributions to clinical trials. American Journal of Epidemiology 104 (1976) 408 - 421

Cornfield, J., W. Haenszel: Some aspects of retrospective studies. Journal of Chronic Diseases 11 (1960) 523 - 534

Feinstein, A.R.: Clinical biostatistics: The epidemiologic trohoc, the relative risk ratio, and retrospective research. Clinical Pharmacology and Therapeutics 14 (1973) 291 - 307

Fink, H.: Grundsätze des kontrollierten Versuchs. Arzneimittelforschung/ Drug Research 28 (1978) 2017 - 2019

Fischer, L., K. Patil: Matching and unirelatedness. American Journal of Epidemiology 100 (1974) 347 - 349

Freedman, R.: Incomplete matching in ex-post facto studies. American Journal of Sociology 55 (1950) 485 - 487

Friebel, H.: Langzeitversuch und Langzeiterfahrung in der angewandten Therapie (Phase IV). In: K.W. Eickstedt, F. Gross (Hrsg.): Klinische Arzneimittelprüfung . Stuttgart: Gustav Fischer 1975, 145 - 151

Gehan, E.A., E.J. Freireich: Non-randomized controls in cancer clinical trials. New England Journal of Medicine 290 (1974) 198 - 203

Gordis, L.: Assuring the quality of questionnaire data in epidemiologic research. American Journal of Epidemiology 109 (1979) 21 - 24

Gordon, T., F.E. Moore, D. Shurtleff, T.R. Dawber: Some methodologic problems in the longterm-study of cardiovascular disease: Observations in the Framingham Study. Journal of Chronic Diseases 10 (1959) 186 - 206

Greenland, S.: Response and follow-up bias in cohort studies. American Journal of Epidemiology 106 (1977) 184 - 187

Gross, F.H., W.H.W. Inman (Eds.): Drug monitoring. New York, London: Academic Press 1977

Hardy, R.H., C. White: Matching in retrospective studies. American Journal of Epidemiology 93 (1971) 75

Harris, E.L., J.D. Fitzgerald (Eds.): The principles and practice of clinical trials. Edinburgh, London : Livingstone 1970

Hill, A.B.: The principles of medical statistics. 8th edition. London : Lancet 1966

Hölzel, D., K. Überla: Grundsätze der Versuchsplanung. In: H.P. Kümmerle (Hrsg.): Methoden der klinischen Pharmakologie. München : Urban & Schearzenberg 1978, 37 - 57

Holford, T.R., C. White, J.L. Kelsey: Multivariate analysis for matched case-control-studies. American Journal of Epidemiology 107 (1978) 245 - 256

Imhof, P.R.: Erwünschte und unerwünschte Wirkungen von Prüfpräparaten bei Phase-I-Studien. Arzneimittelforschung/Drug Research 23 (1973) 1147 - 1152

Jesdinsky, H.J. (Hrsg.): Memorandum zur Planung und Durchführung kontrollierter klinischer Therapiestudien, Schriftenreihe der GMDS, No. 1, Stuttgart : Schattauer 1978

Jesdinsky, H.J.: Planung einer Studie. In: G. Füllgraf, H. Kewitz (Hrsg.): Arzneimittelprüfung durch den niedergelassenen Arzt. Stuttgart : Gustav Fischer 1979, 44 - 59

Jick, H.: The discovery of drug induced illness. New England Journal of Medicine 296 (1977) 481 - 485

Jick, H., M.P. Vessey: Case-control studies in the evaluation of drug induced illness. American Journal of Epidemiology 107 (1978) 1 - 7

Kleinsorge, H.: Problematik der Bewertung experimenteller Voruntersuchungen für die klinische Prüfung neuer Pharmaka. Arzneimittelforschung/Drug Research 25 (1975) 1112 - 1118

Koller, S.: Auswertung. In: S. Koller, G. Wagner (Hrsg.): Handbuch der medizinischen Dokumentation und Datenverarbeitung. Stuttgart : Schattauer 1975, 289 - 317

Lindley, D.V.: Making decisions. New York, London: Wiley 1975

Mantel, N., W. Haenszel: Statistical aspects of the analysis of data from retrospective studies of disease. Journal of the National Cancer Institute 22 (1959) 719 - 748

McKinlay, S.M.: Pair-matching - A reappraisal of a popular technique. Biometrics 33 (1977) 725 - 735

McKinlay, S.M.: The design and analysis of the observational study: A review. Journal of the American Statistical Association 70 (1975) 503 - 520

McKinlay, S.M.: The expected number of matches and its variance, for matched pair designs. Applied Statistics 23 (1974) 372 - 383

MacMahon, B., T.F. Pugh: Epidemiology: Principles and Methods. Boston, Mass.: Little Brown and Company 1970

Meier, P.: Statistics and medical experimentation. Biometrics 31 (1975) 511 - 529

Meydrech, E.F., L.L. Kupper: Cost considerations and sample size requirements in cohort and case control studies. American Journal of Epidemiology 107 (1978) 201 - 205

Miettinen, O.S.: The matched pairs design in the case of all-or-none response. Biometrics 24 (1968) 339 - 352

Miettinen, O.S.: Individual matching with multiple controls in the case of all-or-none response. Biometrics 25 (1969) 339 - 355

Miettinen, O.S.: Estimation of relative risk from individually matched series. Biometrics 26 (1970) 75 - 86

Miettinen, O.S.: Estimability and estimation in case-referent studies. American Journal of Epidemiology 103 (1976) 226 - 235

O'Neil, R.T., C. Anello: Case-control-studies: A sequential approach. American Journal of Epidemiology 108 (1978) 415 - 424

Nüssel, E., F.-J. Hehl, R. Scola: Die Gesamtkonzeption der epidemiologischen Herzinfarktforschung in Heidelberg. Medizinische Technik 95 (1975) 109 - 112

Peto, .R., M.C. Pike, P. Armitage, N.E. Breslow, D.R. Cox, S.V. Howard, N. Mantel, K. McPershon, J. Peto, P.G. Smith: Design and analysis of randomized clinical trials requiring prolonged observation of each patient, Part I. British Journal of Cancer 34 (1976) 585 - 612; Part II: British Journal of Cancer 35 (1977) 1 - 39

Pike, M.C., J. Casagrande, P.G. Smith: Statistical analysis of individually matched case-control studies in epidemiology: Factor under study a discrete variable taking multiple values. British Journal of Preventive and Social Medicine 29 (1975) 196 - 201

Pocock, S.J.: Group sequential methods in the design and analysis of clinical trials. Biometrica 64 (1977) 191 - 199

Prentice, R.: Use of the logistic model in retrospective studies. Biometrics 32 (1976) 599 - 607

Raiffa, H.: Decision analysis: Introductory lectures on choices under uncertainty. Reading, Mass.: Eddison Wesley 1968

Schlesselman, J.J.: Sample size requirements in cohort and case-control studies of disease. American Journal of Epidemiology 99 (1974) 381 - 384

Seigel, D.H., S.W. Greenhouse: Multiple relative risk functions in case-control studies. American Journal of Epidemiology 97 (1973) 324 - 331

Selbmann, H.K.: Grenzen und methodische Schwierigkeiten bei multizentrischen Studien. Arzneimittelforschung/Drug Research 28 (1978) 2023 - 2026

Shapiro, S., D. Slone: Case-control surveillance. In: F.H. Gross, W.H.W. Inman (Eds.): Drug monitoring. London, New York: Academic Press, 1977

Staak, M., A. Weiser: Klinische Prüfung von Arzneimitteln. Methodik und Rechtsgrundlagen. Stuttgart : Enke 1978

Susser, M.: Causal thinking in health sciences: Concepts and strategies in epidemiology. New York: Oxford University Press 1973

Susser, M.: Judgement and causal inference: criteria in epidemiologic studies. American Journal of Epidemiology 105 (1977) 1 - 15

Überla, K.: Versuchsplanung und Statistik in Phase II und III. Arznei-mittelforschung/Drug Research 23 (1973) 1192 - 1196

Überla, K.: Die biometrische Planung und Auswertung klinischer Prüfun-gen. In: K.W. v. Eickstedt, F. Gross (Hrsg.): Klinische Arznei-mittelprüfung. Stuttgart : Gustav Fischer 1975, 137 - 144

Überla, K.: Versuchsplanung in Phase I. Arzneimittelforschung/Drug Re-search 28 (1978) 2032 - 2036

Walter, S.D.: Determination of significant relative risks and optimal sampling procedures in prospective and retrospective comparative studies of various sizes. American Journal of Epidemiology 105 (1977) 387 - 397

Wolf, H.P.: Klinisch -chemische Untersuchungen in Phase I der Arznei-mittelprüfung am Menschen. Arzneimittelforschung/Drug Research 25 (1975) 1124 - 1126

Worcester, J.: Matched samples in epidemiologic studies. Biometrics 20 (1964) 840 - 848

Chapter 2

Ambler, S.: Statistical analysis of clinical trial data. In: F.N. John-son, S. Johnson (Eds.): Clinical Trials. Oxford: Blackwell 1977, 83 - 107

Armitage, P.: Sequential medical trials. Oxford: Blackwell 1975

Bearman, J.E.: Writing the protocol for a clinical trial . American Journal of Ophtalmology 79 (1975) 775 - 778

Bennet, A.E., K. Ritchie: Questionnaires in medicine - A guide to their design and use. London: Oxford University Press 1975

Bentel, P., H. Kuffner, E. Röck, W. Schubö: SPSS - Statistik Programm-system für die Sozialwissenschafren nach NIE, HULL, JENKINS, STEINBRENNER, BENT. Stuttgart: Gustav Fischer 1980

Berdie, D.R., J.F. Anderson: Questionnaires, design and use. Metuchen, N.Y.: Scarecrow Press 1974

Berger, P.M., R.A. Stallones: Legal Liability and epidemiologic research. American Journal of Epidemiology 106 (1977) 177 - 183

Breslow, N.: Perspectives on the statistician's role in cooperative clinical research. Cancer 41 (1978) 326 - 332

Bross, I.D.J.: Sequential medical plans. Biometrics 8 (1952) 188 - 205

Bulpitt, C.J.: The design of clinical trials. British Journal of Hospi-tal Medicine 13 (1975) 611 - 680

Burley, D.M.: Designing the correct protocol. In: C.S. Good (Ed.): The principles and practice of clinical trials. Edinburgh: Churchill Livingstone 1976

Byar, D.P., R.M. Simon, W.T. Friedewald, J.J. Schlesselman, D.L. De Mets, J.H. Ellenberg, M.H. Gail, J.H. Ware: Randomized clinical trials. New England Journal of Medicine 295 (1976) 74 - 80

Carter, S.K.: Clinical trials in cancer chemotherapy. Cancer 40 (1977) 544 - 557

Chalmers, T.C., J.B. Block, S. Lee: Controlled studies in clinical can-cer research. New England Journal of Medicine 287 (1972) 75 - 78

Clark, C.J., C.C. Downie: A method for the rapid determination of the number of patients to include in a controlled clinical trial. Lancet 2 (1966) 1357 - 1358

Cornfield, J.: Recent methodological contributions to clinical trials. American Journal of Epidemiology 104 (1976) 408 - 421

Cranston, W.I., G.E. Sowton, J.D. Fitzgerald: Cardiovascular drug evaluation. In: E.L. Harris, J.D. Fitzgerald (Eds.): The principles and practice of clinical trials. London, Edinburgh: Livingstone 1970, 134 - 164

Daniel, G.R., M. Shephard, M. Hamilton : Evaluation of psychotropic drugs. In: E.L. Harris, J.D. Fitzgerald (Eds.): The principles and practice of clinical trials. London, Edinburgh: Livingstone 1970, 189 - 226

Deeley, T.J.: The random allocation of patients in clinical trials. Methods of Information in Medicine 5 (1966) 100 - 101

Dixon, W.J. (Ed.): BMDP Biomedical computer programs. Berkeley: Universtiy of California Press 1981

Documenta Geigy: Wissenschaftliche Tabellen. Stuttgart : Thieme 1975

Ederer, P.: Practical problems in collaborative clinical trials. American Journal of Epidemiology 102 (1975) 111 - 118

von Eickstedt, K.W., F. Gross (Hrsg.): Klinische Arzneimittelprüfung. Stuttgart : Gustav Fischer 1975

van Eimeren, W., K. Überla: Thesen zu Problemen des Arzneimittelrechts aus statistischer und methodischer Sicht. Pharma Dialog 36 (1975) 3 - 17

Feinstein, A.R.: Clinical biostatistics. Saint Louis: Mosby Company 1977

Feinstein, A.R.: Clinical biostatistics XXII - XXIV, The role of randomization in sampling, testing, allocation, and credulous idolatry. Clinical Pharmacology and Therapeutics 14 (1973) 601 - 615, 898 - 915, 1035 - 1051

Feinstein, A.R., J.R. Landis: The role of prognostic stratification in preventing the bias permitted by random allocation of treatment. Journal of Chronic Diseases 29 (1976) 277 - 284

Fink, H.: Zur Frage der Zahl der Probanden oder Patienten in klinisch-pharmakologischen Studien. International Journal of Clinical Pharmacology 14 (1976) 66 - 74

Flamant, R. (Ed.): Controlled therapeutic trials in cancer. UICC Technical Report Series, Vol. 8. Genf: UICC 1972

Fülgraff, G., H. Kewitz (Hrsg.): Arzneimittelprüfung durch den niedergelassenen Arzt. Stuttgart : Gustav Fischer 1979

Galbraith, A.W.: Getting the trial off the ground: logistics, presentation of supplies. In: C.S. Good (Ed.): The principles and practice of clinical trials. Edinburgh: Livingstone 1976, 101 - 106

Gehan, E.A., E.J. Freireich: Non-randomized controls in cancer clinical trials. New England Journal of Medicine 290 (1974) 198 - 203

George, S.L., M.M. Desu: Planning the size and duration of a clinical trial studying the time to some clinical event. Journal of Chronic Diseases 27 (1974) 15 - 24

Good, C.S. (Ed.): The principles and practice of clinical trials. Edinburgh: Churchill Livingstone 1976

Gordis, L.: Assuring the quality of questionnaire data in epidemiologic research. American Journal of Epidemiology 109 (1979) 21 - 24

Grady, F.: Designing the report form. In: Good, C.S. (Ed.): The principles and practice of clinical trials. Edinburgh: Livingstone 1976, 60 - 74

Grady, F.: Handling data of trial results. C.S. Good (Ed.): The principles and practice of clinical trials. Edinburgh: Livingstone 1976, 122 - 128

Green, S.B., D.P. Byar: The effect of stratified randomization on size and power of statistical tests in clinical trials. Journal of Chronic Diseases 31 (1978) 445 - 454

Grimshaw, J.J.: Statistical analysis of trial results. C.S. Good (Ed.): The principles and practice of clinical trials. Edinburgh: Livinstone 1976, 129 - 137

Grizzle, J.E.: The case for management research for large field trials. Journal of Chronic Diseases 30 (1977) 257 - 259

Halperin, M., E. Rogot, J. Gurian, F. Ederer: Sample sizes for medical trials with special reference to long-term therapy. Journal of Chronic Diseases 21 (1968) 13 - 24

Harris, E.L., J.D. Fitzgerald (Eds.): The principles and practice of clinical trials. Edinburgh, London: Livingstone 1970

Hasskarl, H.: Rechtliche Zulässigkeit der klinischen Prüfung. Deutsches Ärzteblatt 75 (1978) 1087 - 1094 und 1150 - 1155

Hasskarl, H., H. Kleinsorge: Arzneimittelprüfung - Arzneimittelrecht. Stuttgart : Gustav Fischer 1979

Hawkins, C.F.: Presentation of results. In: C.S. Good (Ed.): The principles and practice of clinical trials. Edinburgh: 1976, 138 - 146

Hölzel, D., K. Überla: Grundsätze der Versuchsplanung. In: H.P. Kuemmerle (Hrsg.): Methoden der klinischen Pharmakologie. München : Urban und Schwarzenberg 1978, 37 - 57

Huskisson, E.C.: Trials of anti-rheumatics drugs. In: C.S. Good (Ed.): The principles and practice of clinical trials. Edinburgh: 1976, 188 - 194

Immich, H.: Praktische Anwendung der Klassifikations- und Codierungsprinzipien. In: S. Koller, G. Wagner (Hrsg.): Handbuch der medizinischen Dokumentation und Datenverarbeitung. Stuttgart : Schattauer 1975, 246 - 266

Jesdinsky, H.J. (Hrsg.): Memorandum zur Planung und Durchführung kontrollierter klinischer Therapiestudien. Schriftenreihe der Deutschen Gesellschaft für Medizinische Dokumentation, Informatik und Statistik. Stuttgart : Schattauer 1978

Jesdinsky, H.J.: Planung einer Studie. In: G. Fülgraff, H. Kewitz (Hrsg.): Arzneimittelprüfung durch den niedergelassenen Arzt. Stuttgart : Gustav Fischer 1979, 44 - 59

Jesdinsky, H.J.: Statistische Auswertung. In: G. Fülgraff, H. Kewitz (Hrsg.): Arzneimittelprüfung durch den niedergelassenen Arzt. Stuttgart : Gustav Fischer 1979, 96 - 123

Johnson, F.N., S. Johnson (Eds.): Clinical trials. Oxford: Blackwell 1977

Johnson, F.N., S. Johnson: Organisation of clinical trials. In: F.N. Johnson, S. Johnson (Eds.): Clinical trials. Oxford: Blackwell 1977, 36 - 82

Kempthorne, O.: Of what use are tests of significance and tests of hypothesis. Communications of Statistical Theory and Methodology 8 (1976) 763 - 777

Kempthorne, O.: Why randomize? Journal of Statistical Planning and Inference 1 (1977) 1 - 25

Köhler, C.O.: Datenverarbeitungsanlagen. In: S. Koller, G. Wagner (Hrsg.) Handbuch der medizinischen Dokumentation und Datenverarbeitung. Stuttgart : Schattauer 1975a, 93 - 117

Köhler, C.O.: Informationsträger. In: S. Koller, G. Wagner (Hrsg.): Handbuch der medizinischen Dokumentation und Datenverarbeitung. Stuttgart : Schattauer 1975b, 11 - 28

Köpcke, W., K. Überla: Dokumentation und Datenverarbeitung. In: H.P. Kümmerle (Hrsg.): Methoden der Klinischen Pharmakologie. München: Urban & Schwarzenberg 1978, 83 - 99

Koller, S.: Auswertung. In: S. Koller, G. Wagner (Hrsg.): Handbuch der medizinischen Dokumentation und Datenverarbeitung. Stuttgart : Schattauer 1975, 289 - 317

Koller, S., G. Wagner (Hrsg.): Handbuch der medizinischen Dokumentation und Datenverarbeitung. Stuttgart : Schattauer 1975

Kuemmerle, H.P. (Hrsg.): Methoden der klinischen Pharmakologie. München: Urban & Schwarzenberg 1978

Lawrie, T.D.V., W.S. Hillis, A. Tweddel: Anti-anginal trials. In: C.S. Good (Ed.): The principles and practice of clinical trials. Edinburgh: Lvingstone 1976, 153 - 162

Levy, P.M.: Interpretation of clinical trials. In: F.N. Johnson, S. Johnson (Eds.): Clinical trials. Oxford: Blackwell 1977, 129 - 146

Lewandowski, G.: Rechtliche Voraussetzungen.In: G. Fülgraff, H. Kewitz (Hrsg.): Arzneimittelprüfung durch den niedergelassenen Arzt. Stuttgart : Gustav Fischer 1979, 10 - 17

Liberman, R.: An analysis of the placebo phenomenon. Journal of Chronic Diseases 15 (1961) 761 - 783

Marsh, B.T.: Keeping the trial going: Medical advisers or coordinators: Prescription costs. In: C.S. Good (Ed.): The principles and practice of clinical trials. Edinburgh: Livingstone 1976, 107 - 114

Martini, P., G. Oberhoffer, E. Welte: Methodenlehre der therapeutisch-klinischen Forschung. Berlin : Springer 1968

Maxwell, C.: The significance of significance. Clinical Trials Journal 5 (1968) 1015 - 1020

Maxwell, C.: The choice of design for clinical trials. Clinical Trials Journal 5 (1968) 1139 - 1143

May, W.W.: The composition and function of ethical committees. Journal of Medical Ethics 1 (1975) 23 - 29

McKinlay, S.M.: Pair matching - A reappraisal of a popular technique. Biometrics 33 (1977) 725 - 735

McPershon, K.: Sequential analysis in clinical trials. In: F.N. Johnson, S. Johnson (Eds.): Clinical Trials. Oxford: Blackwell 1977, 108 - 128

Meier, P.: Statistics and medical experimentation. Biometrics 31 (1975) 511 - 529

Meydrech, E.F., L.L. Kuuper: Cost considerations and sample size requirements in cohort and case-control studies. American Journal of Epidemiology 107 (1978) 201 - 2o5

Müller-Römer, D.: Arzneimittelrecht von A - Z. Neu-Isenburg/München: Otto Hoffmann 1978

Nicholson, P.A.: Budgeting for clinical trials. In: C.S. Good (Ed.): The principles and practice of clinical trials. Edinburgh: Livingstone 1976, 81 - 86

O'Fallon, J.R., S.D. Dubey, D.S. Salsburg, J.H. Edmonson, A. Soffer, T. Colton: Should there be statistical guidelines for medical research papers. Biometrics 34 (1978) 687 - 695

Peto, R., M.C. Pike, P. Armitage, N.E. Breslow, D.R. Cow, S.V. Howard, N. Mantel, K. McPherson, J. Peto, P.G. Smith: Design and analysis of randomized clinical trials requiring prolonged observation of each patient, I.Introduction and design. British Journal of Cancer 34 (1976) 585 - 612, II. Analysis and example. British Journal of Cancer 35 (1977) 1 - 39

Pocock, S.J.: The combination of randomized and historical controls in clinical trials. Journal of Chronic Diseases 29 (1976) 175 - 188

Proppe, A.: Datenerfassung. In: S. Koller, G. Wagner (Hrsg.): Handbuch der medizinischen Dokumentation und Datenverarbeitung. Stuttgart: Schattauer 1975, 199 - 211

Revidierte Deklaration von Helsinki:"Empfehlung für Ärzte, die in der biomedizinischen Forschung am Menschen tätig sind", beschlossen von der 29. Generalversammlung des Weltärztebundes am 10. Oktober 1975 in Tokio, Deutsches Ärzteblatt 72 (1975) 3162 - 3163

Robinson, B.N.: SIR - Scientific Information Retrieval - User's Manual. SIR Incorp. Evanston. Ill.: 1980

Rudnick, S., R.L. Capizzi: The conduct of therapeutic trials in cancer medicine. Seminars in Oncology 4 (1977) 255 - 258

Sachs, L.: Angewandte Statistik. Berlin : Springer 1978

SAS-Institute: SAS User's Guide. SAS Incorp. Cary N.C.: 1981

Schindel, L.: Placebo and Placeboeffekte in Klinik und Forschung. Arzneimittelforschung 17 (1967) 892 - 918

Schlesselman, J.J.: Sample size requirements in cohort and case-control studies of disease. American Journal of Epidemiology 99 (1974) 381 - 384

Schneidermann, M.A.: The proper size of clinical trials : "Grandma's strudel method". Journal of New Drugs 4 (1964) 3 - 11

Schnieders, B.: Organisatorische Voraussetzunge. In: G. Fülgraff, H. Kewitz (Hrsg.): Arzneimittelprüfung durch den niedergelassenen Arzt. Stuttgart : Gustav Fischer 1979, 18 - 25

Schork, M.H., R.Remington: Determination for sample size in treatment - control comparison for chronic disease studies in which dropout or non-adherence give a problem. Journal of Chronic Diseases 20 (1967) 233 - 239

Schwartz, W.B. G.A. Gorry, J.P. Kasirer, A. Essig: Decision analysis and clinical judgment. American Journal of Medicine 55 (1974) 459 - 472

Selbmann, H.K.: Statistische Auswertungsverfahren in der klinisch-therapeutischen Forschung. In: H.P. Kuemmerle (Hrsg.): Methoden der klinischen Pharmakologie. München: Urban und Schwarzenberg 1978, 59 - 82

Selbmann, H.K.: Grenzen und methodische Schwierigkeiten bei multizentrischen Studien. Arzneimittelforschung/Drug Research 28 (1978) 2023 - 2026

Smith, R.N.: Ethical aspects of drug evaluation. In: F.N. Johnson, S. Johnson (Eds.): Clinical Trials. Oxford: Blackwell 1977, 162 - 175

Snell, E.S.: The choice of investigator. In: C.S. Good (Ed.): The principles and practice of clinical trials. Edinburgh: Livingstone 1976, 75 - 80

Sondik, E.J. B.W. Brown, A. Silvers: High risk subjects and the cost of large field trials. Journal of Chronic Diseases 27 (2974) 177 - 187

Staak, M., A. Weiser: Klinische Prüfung von Arzneimitteln - Methodik und Rechtsgrundlagen. Stuttgart : Enke 1978

Tancredi, L.R.: The ethics quagmire and random clinical trials. Inquiry 12 (1975) 171 - 179

Überla, K.: Die biometrische Planung und Auswertung klinischer Prüfungen. In: K.W. von Eickstedt, F. Gross (Hrsg.): Klinische Arzneimittelprüfung. Stuttgart : Gustav Fischer 1975, 137 - 144

Wade, P.: Information retrieval. In: E.L. Harris, J.D. Fitzgerald (Eds.): The principles and practice of clinical trials. London, Edinburgh: Livingstone 1970, 37 - 40

Wagner, G.: Datenkontrolle. In: S. Koller, G. Wagner (Hrsg.): Handbuch der medizinischen Dokumentation und Datenverarbeitung. Stuttgart: Schattauer 1975, 267 - 288

Walter, E. (Hrsg.): Statistische Methoden I, Grundlagen der Versuchsplanung. Berlin : Springer 1970

Weinstein, M.C.: Allocation of subjects in medical experiments. New England Journal of Medicine 291 (1974) 1278 - 1285

Wittenborn, J.R. (Ed.): Guidelines for clinical trials of psychotropic drugs. Pharmakopsychiatrie/Neuro-Psychopharmakologie 10 (1977) 205 - 231

World Health Organization: Principles for the clinical evaluation of drugs. Technical Report Series 403, 1968

World Health Organization: Guidelines for evaluation of drugs for use in man. Technical Report Series 563, 1975

Zelen, M.: The randomization and stratification of patients to clinical trials. Journal of Chronic Diseases 27 (1974) 365 - 375

Zelen, M.: Aspects of the planning and analysis of clinical trials in cancer. In: J.N. Srivastava (Ed.): A Survey of Statistical Design and Linear Models. Amsterdam: North Holland 1975, 629 - 646

Zelen, M.: Statistical options in clinical trials. Seminars in Oncology 4 (1977) 441 - 446

Chapter 3

Agras, St., G. Marshall: Recruitment for the coronary primary prevention trial. In: H.P. Roth, R.S. Gordon (Eds.): Proceedings of the National Conference on Clinical Trials Methodology. Clinical Pharmacology and Therapeutics 25 (1979) 688 - 690

Bundesärztekammer (Hrsg.): Prüfung neuer Arzneimittel in der Praxis des niedergelassenen Arztes. Deutsches Ärzteblatt 75 (1978) 2773 - 2778

Croke, G.: Recruitment for the National Cooperative Gallstone Study. In: H.P. Roth, R.S. Gordon (Eds.): Proceedings of the National

Conference on Clinical Trials Methodology. Clinical Pharmacology and Therapeutics 25 (1979) 691 - 694

Dreher , R.: Gründe für nur mangelhafte kontrollierte Therapiestudien in der Rheumatologie. In: ISR (Internationales Institut für wissenschaftliche Zusammenarbeit e.V. Schloß Reisensburg) (Hrsg.): Probleme und Randbedingungen von Therapiestudien, Methodenkolloquium I, Schloß Reisensburg, 27. - 29. April 1978, 112 - 115

Evans, J.T.: Internal monitoring: Patient and study management at the clinic. In: H.P. Roth, R.S. Gordon (Eds.): Proceedings of the National Conference on Clinical Trials Methodology. Clinical Pharmacology and Therapeutics 25 (1979) 712 - 716

Grimm, R.H., K. Shimoni, W.R. Harlan, E.H. Estes: Evaluation of patient-care protocol use by various providers. New England Journal of Medicine 292 (1975) 507 - 511

Hagans, J.: The design and methodology of cooperative drug trials. Drug Intelligence and Clinical Pharmacy 8 (1974) 531 - 534

Kahn, H.A., H. Leibowitz, J.P. Ganley, M. Kini, Th. Colton, R. Nickerson, T.R. Dawber: Standardizing diagnostic procedures. American Journal of Opthalmology 79 (1975) 768 - 775

Klimt, P., P.C. Canner : Terminating a long-term clinical trial. In : H.P. Roth, R.S. Gordon (Eds.): Proceedings of the National Conference on Clinical Trials Methodology. Clinical Pharmacology and Therapeutics 29 (1979) 641 - 646

Meier, P.: Terminating a trial - the ethicàl problem. In: H.P. Roth, R.S. Gordon (Eds.): Proceedings of the National Conference on Clinical Trials Methodology. Clinical Pharmacology and Therapeutics 25 (1979) 633 - 640

Mowery, R.L., Williams, D.P.: Aspects of clinic monitoring in large-scale multiclinic trials. In: H.P. Roth, R.S. Gordon (Eds.): Proceedings of the National Conference on Clinical Trials Methodology. Clinical Pharmacology and Therapeutics 29 (1979) 717 - 719

Schreml, W.: Diskussion der Methodik von Therapiestudien im Bereich Krebs anhand von zwei Beispielen : Melanom- und Mamma-Carcinom-Studie. In: ISR (Hrsg.): Probleme und Randbedingungen von Therapiestudien, Methodenkolloquium I, Schloß Reisensburg, 27. - 29. April 1978, 43 - 53

Stauch, M.: Herz-Kreislauf-Therapiestudien in USA und in der Bundesrepublik. In: ISR (Hrsg.): Probleme und Randbedingungen von Therapiestudien, Methodenkolloquium I, Schloß Reisensburg, 27. - 29. April 1978, 81 - 86

Williams, O.D.: A framework for quality assurance of clinical data. In: H.P. Roth, R.S. Gordon (Eds.): Proceedings of the National Conference on Clinical Trials Methodology. Clinical Pharmacology and Therapeutics 29 (1979) 700 - 702

Chapter 4

Benkert, O.: Forschungsansätze bei psycho-pharmakologischen Studien. In: ISR (Hrsg.): Probleme und Randbedingungen von Therapiestudien, Methodenkolloqium II. Schloß Reisensburg, 29. - 30. Juni 1978, 65 - 73

Blalock, H.M.: Measurement in the social sciences. Chicago: Aldine 1974

Brook, R.H., A. Davies-Avery, S. Greenfield, L.J. Harris, T. Lelak, N.E. Solomon, J.E. Ware : Assessing the quality of medical care using outcome measures: An overview of the method. Medical Care Supplement 15, 1977

Brook, R.H., J.E. Ware, A. Davies-Avery, A.L. Stewart, C.A. Donald, W.H. Rogers, K.N. Williams, S.A. Johnston: Conceptualization and measurement of health for adults in the Health Insurance Study: Vol. VIII Overview. Santa Monica, Ca.: Rand R-1987/8 HEW, October 1979

CIPS (Collegium Internationale Psychiatriae Scalarum) (Hrsg.): Internationale Skalen für Psychiatrie. Weinheim: Beltz 1981

Donald, C.A., J.E. Ware, R.H. Brook, A. Davies-Avery: Conceptualization and measurement of health for adults in the Health Insurance Study: Vol. IV, Social health. Santa Monica, Ca.: Rand R-1987/4 HEW, August 1978

Guttentag, M., E.L. Struening (Eds.): Handbook of evaluation research. London: Sage 1975

NCHS (National Center of Health Statistics) (Ed.): Clearinghouse on health indexes, Bibliography quarterly since 1973

Stewart, A.L., J.E. Ware, R.H. Brook, A. Dvaies-Avery: Conceptualization and measurement of health for adults in the Health Insurance Study: Vol. II, Physical health in terms of functioning. Santa Monica, Ca.: Rand R-1987/2 - HEW, July 1978

Ströbel, G.: Einzelprobleme bei Therapiestudien über rheumatische Arthritis und chronische Polyarthritis. In: ISR (Hrsg.): Probleme und Randbedingungen von Therapiestudien, Methodenkolloquium I, Schloß Reisensburg, 29. - 30. Juni 1978, 105 - 111

Ware, J.E., S.A. Johnston, A. Davies-Avery, R.H. Brook: Conceptualization and measurement of health for adults in the Health Insurance Study: Vol. III, Mental health. Santa Monica, Ca.: Rand R-1987/3-HEW, Dezember 1979

Ware, J.E., R.H. Brook, A. Davies-Avery, K.N. Williams, A.L. Stewart, W.H. Rogers, C.A. Donald, S.A. Johnston: Conceptualization and measurement of health for adults in the Health Insurance Study: Vol. I, Model of health and methodology. Santa Monica, Ca.: Rand R-1987/1-HEW, May 1980

Chapter 5

Bar, Ch. von, G. Fischer: Haftung bei der Planung und Förderung medizinischer Forschungsvorhaben. Neue juristische Wochenschrift 50 (1980) 2734 - 2740

BMFT (Bundesministerium für Forschung und Technologie) (Hrsg.): The Federal Government's Program on Promoting Research and Development in the Service of Health 1978 - 1981, Bonn : 1978

Chalmers, Th.C.: The ethics of randomization as a decision making technique and the problem of informed consent. USDHEW Report of the 14th annual Conference of Cardiovascular Training Grant Program Directors. National Heart Institute, 1967

Chalmers, Th.C.: Randomization of the first patient. Medical Clinics of North-America 59 (1975) 1035 - 1038

Cochrane, A.L.: Effectiveness and efficiency. London : The Nuffield Provincial Hospital Trust,1972

Deutsch, E.: Das Recht der klinischen Forschung am Menschen. Frankfurt: Lang 1979

Fletscher, J.C.: Realities of patient consent to medical research. Hastings Center Studies 1 (1973) 39 - 49

Freireich, E.J., E.A. Gehan: The limitations of the randomized clinical
    trial. In: V.T. de Vita, H. Busch (Eds.): Cancer drug development.
    New York: Academic Press 1979, 277 - 310

Hasskarl, H., H. Kleinsorge : Arzneimittelprüfung - Arzneimittelrecht.
    Stuttgart : Gustav Fischer 1979

Helmchen, H., B. Müller-Oerlinghausen (Hrsg.): Psychiatrische Therapie-
    forschung. Ethische und juristische Probleme. Berlin, Heidelberg,
    New York : Springer 1978

Lasagna, L.: Problems in publication of clinical trial methodology. In:
    H.P. Roth, R.S. Gordon (Eds.): Proceedings of the National Con-
    ference on Clinical Trials Methodology. Clinical Pharmacology and
    Therapeutics 25 (1979) 751 - 753

Levine, R.J., K. Lebacqz: Some ethical considerations in clinical
    trials. In : H.P. Roth, R.S. Gordon (Eds.): Proceedings of the
    National Conference on Clinical Trials Methodology. Clinical
    Pharmacology and Therapeutics 25 (1979) 728 - 741

Lewandowski, G.: Rechtliche Voraussetzungen. In: G. Fülgraff, A. Kewitz
    (Hrsg.): Arzneimittelprüfung durch den niedergelassenen Arzt.
    Stuttgart :Thieme 1979, 10 - 17

Linzbach, M.: Informed consent - Die Aufklärungspflicht des Arztes im
    amerikanischen und deutschen Recht. Frankfurt : Lang 1980

Meinert, C.L.: Toward more definitive clinical trials. Paper prepared
    for the National Commission on Digestive Diseases through a work
    group of the Subcommittee on Research - Targeted and Nondirected,
    1978

Meinert, C.L., B.S. Hawkins: Methodology : The case of improved commu-
    nications. In: H.P. Roth, R.S. Gordon (Eds.): Proceedings of the
    National Conference on Clinical Trials Methodology. Clinical
    Pharmacology and Therapeutics 25 (1979) 754 - 757

Mosteller, F.: Problems of omission in communications. In: H.P. Roth,
    R.S. Gordon (Eds.): Proceedings of the National Conference on
    Clinical Trials Methodology. Clinical Pharmacology and Therapeu-
    tics 25 (1979) 761 - 766

Relman, A.S.: Publications and promotions for the clinical investiga-
    tor. in: H.P. Roth, R.S. Gordon (Eds.): Proceedings of the Na-
    tional Conference on Clinical Trials Methodology. Clinical Phar-
    macology and Therapeutics 25 (1979) 673 - 678

Roth, H.P., R.S. Gordon (Eds.): Proceedings of the National Conference
    on Clinical Trials Methodology. Clinical Pharmacology and Thera-
    peutics 25 (1979)

Schoolman, H.M.: Retrieving information on clinical trial methodology.
    In: H.P. Roth, R.S. Gordon (Eds.): Proceedings of the National
    Conference on Clinical Trials Methodology. Clinical Pharmacology
    and Therapeutics 25 (1979) 758 - 760

Medizinische Informatik und Statistik